Joint Review of the Cambodian National Health Sector Response to HIV 2013

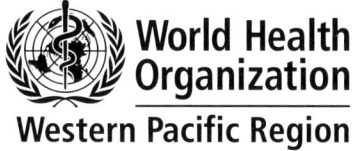

WHO Library Cataloguing-in-Publication Data

Joint review of the Cambodian national health sector response to HIV 2013

1. AIDS-related opportunistic infections – prevention and control. 2. HIV infections – prevention and control. 3. National health programs – Cambodia.
I. World Health Organization Regional Office for the Western Pacific

ISBN 978 92 9061 664 1   (NLM Classification: WC 503)

© World Health Organization 2014

All rights reserved. Publications of the World Health Organization are available on the WHO website (www.who.int) or can be purchased from WHO Press, World Health Organization, 20 Avenue Appia, 1211 Geneva 27, Switzerland (tel.: +41 22 791 3264; fax: +41 22 791 4857;
e-mail: bookorders@who.int).

Requests for permission to reproduce or translate WHO publications –whether for sale or for non-commercial distribution– should be addressed to WHO Press through the WHO website (www.who.int/about/licensing/copyright_form/en/index.html). For WHO Western Pacific Regional Publications, request for permission to reproduce should be addressed to Publications Office, World Health Organization, Regional Office for the Western Pacific, P.O. Box 2932, 1000, Manila, Philippines, fax: +632 521 1036, e-mail: publications@wpro.who.int

The designations employed and the presentation of the material in this publication do not imply the expression of any opinion whatsoever on the part of the World Health Organization concerning the legal status of any country, territory, city or area or of its authorities, or concerning the delimitation of its frontiers or boundaries. Dotted lines on maps represent approximate border lines for which there may not yet be full agreement.

The mention of specific companies or of certain manufacturers' products does not imply that they are endorsed or recommended by the World Health Organization in preference to others of a similar nature that are not mentioned. Errors and omissions excepted, the names of proprietary products are distinguished by initial capital letters.

All reasonable precautions have been taken by the World Health Organization to verify the information contained in this publication. However, the published material is being distributed without warranty of any kind, either expressed or implied. The responsibility for the interpretation and use of the material lies with the reader. In no event shall the World Health Organization be liable for damages arising from its use.

Table of contents

Acknowledgements	iv
Executive summary	v
Acronyms	vii
Introduction	1
Status and trends of HIV in Cambodia and responses to the epidemics	3
Findings and recommendations	10
1. Policy, strategy and structures	10
2. Creating an enabling environment	14
3. Strategic information	16
4. Maintaining control of the epidemic	24
5. Optimizing the cascade of interventions: HIV testing, linkages to prevention, care and treatment	35
6. Tuberculosis and HIV	51
7. HIV/STI laboratory services	54
8. Pharmaceutical supply management	56
9. Blood safety	64
10. Sustainable financing for the HIV/AIDS response	65
General conclusions and summary	69
References	73
Annex I: Review team members	76
Annex II: Overall schedule, scope and process of national health sector review	77
Annex III: Programme of work and assignments	81
Annex IV: Meetings and visits to institutions in Phnom Penh	83
Annex V: Summary of recommendations	86

Acknowledgements

The members of the joint review team wish to express their gratitude to His Excellency Dr Mam Bun Heng, Minister of Health of the Royal Government of Cambodia, for inviting them to assess the progress achieved by the national health sector response to HIV and sexually transmitted infections in Cambodia. The review team is indebted to the Director, senior staff and personnel of the National Center for HIV/AIDS, Dermatology and STDs for the time and energy they devoted throughout the review process to provide the team with quality information. They facilitated all interviews and communication and, in general, ensured smooth implementation of the review activity. The review team wishes to thank warmly other entities within the Ministry of Health and other ministries for providing it with excellent information and welcoming its visits to their offices and facilities. The review team members express their gratitude to the members of the Steering Committee who provided directions for the review as well as to governmental and nongovernmental partners who have been contributing in a major way to the Cambodian response to HIV. A special note of encouragement goes to the thousands of health workers who are doing a fabulous job across the country, often with insufficient means and little or no personal incentive. Finally, the team acknowledges the resilience, courage, kindness and openness of the members of HIV-affected communities in the country, in particular, the people living with HIV, and wishes them more power in their bold confrontation with the HIV epidemic.

This report was written by Daniel Tarantola, Richard Steen, Jerry Owen Jacobsen and Ying-Ru Lo with contributions from the members of the international and national review teams and secretariat, and under oversight of the Steering Committee and the National Center for HIV/AIDS, Dermatology and STDs manager and staff. The World Health Organization's in-country HIV unit and the National Center for HIV/AIDS, Dermatology and STDs ensured accuracy of the data and review findings, and provided essential administrative and logistic support during the review and while preparing this report.

Finally, the review, development and publication of this report were supported by generous financial contributions from the Global Fund to Fight AIDS, Tuberculosis and Malaria, with additional support through the World Health Organization's HIV & STI unit, Division of Combating Communicable Diseases, Regional Office for the Western Pacific, Manila and the Department of HIV/AIDS, Geneva.

Executive summary

A review of the national health sector response to HIV and sexually transmitted infections (STIs) in Cambodia was conducted from 30 April to 10 May 2013 by a composite team of national and external members. A brief desk review of the impact of the national response to HIV, conducted in January 2013 by two members of the Global Fund to Fight AIDS, Tuberculosis and Malaria and World Health Organization (WHO) team also fed into this activity. The purpose of the review was to assess the progress made under the Strategic Plan for HIV/ AIDS and STI Prevention and Care in Health Sector, 2011–2015. The review focused on the period from 2011 to 2012, and took place at a time when a new conceptual framework for elimination of new HIV infections in Cambodia by 2020 ("Cambodia 3.0") was being finalized. The review team was invited by the leadership of the National Center for HIV/AIDS, Dermatology and STDs (NCHADS) to examine and comment on the contents and feasibility of the new framework.

A locally established steering committee provided a list of issues perceived as particularly relevant to the review. Although the list offered a comprehensive scope for the review, it was eventually abridged by the team, taking into account the following: limited availability of expertise and time, and the pre-existing (or imminent) conduct of focused evaluations and studies on specific topics. During the 10 working days of the review, numerous documents were examined, a series of interviews and observations conducted, and site visits undertaken to governmental and nongovernmental offices, institutions, health structures and community-based services. These activities took place in the municipality of Phnom Penh and in the provinces of Battambang, Banteay Meanchey and Svay Rieng.

The review concluded that the national health sector response to HIV in Cambodia was strong, efficiently directed and managed, and appropriately structured. It recognized opportunities for and obstacles to further progress, as well as how to make more efficient use of available resources. Epidemiological and behavioural evidence suggests that combined prevention, care and treatment efforts have had a positive impact on the epidemic. An abundant number of strategic frameworks, implementation plans, standard operating procedures and guidelines of various types frame the health sector response to HIV. It is supported by a large number of monitoring tools, periodic evaluations and occasional studies. Its strategic design and implementation are guided strongly by a combination of locally produced evidence and international norms, as well as standards and guidance. Altogether, these features place Cambodia's response to HIV as being among the most effective in the world.

The review team concluded that the Cambodian response to HIV was progressing well towards its 2011–2015 strategic objectives, and that it was on track for eliminating the transmission of HIV by 2020 if the following conditions are met:

- Structures, capacities and services dedicated to HIV and STI prevention, care and treatment, and the early diagnosis and treatment of HIV/tuberculosis coinfection are further strengthened and sustained.
- Access to services by the most vulnerable and key affected populations (including entertainment workers, female and male sex workers, men who have sex with men, transsexual and transgender persons and drug users) is expanded and, in some cases, revitalized in a supportive legal and policy environment.

- Stronger follow-up is conducted along the cascade of services, from creation of and demand for voluntary HIV testing and counselling to sustained and efficiently monitored use of care and treatment, devoting particular attention to gender issues, age and key-affected populations. These efforts could be considerably strengthened through effective and better strategic information management, linkage of databases, and tighter communication and collaboration among service providers.
- Sharper epidemiological targeting and more effective interventions are introduced at sufficient intensity and scale to identify new HIV infections and introduce treatment earlier to harness the dual benefit of mortality reduction and prevention of further spread of HIV among those at highest risk.
- Access to, and voluntary use of, HIV counselling and testing by pregnant women attending antenatal clinics is expanded, with full and timely provision of antiretroviral therapy for life during pregnancy and/or shortly before delivery to protect offspring from HIV infection.
- Stronger synergy is fostered within the health sector and across other sectors of development.
- Greater support is provided to health personnel through improved salary, skills upgradation and incentives to ensure staff retention. The health of the Cambodian population is ensured and protected against brain drain and the loss of those who care for them.
- Sustained external financing is assured and a growing financial share secured from national sources.

The review team formulated a series of specific recommendations which, if implemented with a sustained sense of urgency and bolstered by the needed human and financial resources, should enable Cambodia to achieve elimination of new HIV infections by 2020.

Acronyms

3TC	lamivudine
AIDS	acquired immunodeficiency syndrome
ART	antiretroviral therapy
ARV	antiretroviral
AZT	zidovudine
BSS	behavioural surveillance survey
CD4	lymphocyte count (CD4 subgroup) used to monitor HIV progression
CDC	(US) Centers for Disease Control and Prevention
CENAT	National Center for TB and Leprosy Control
CHAI	Clinton Health Access Initiative
CMS	Central Medical Store
CoC	continuum of care
CoPCT	continuum of prevention to care and treatment
CQI	continuous quality improvement
d4T	stavudine
ddI	didanosine
DOT	directly observed treatment, short-course
EFV	efavirenz
ELISA	enzyme-linked immunosorbent assay
EQAS	external quality assurance system
EWI	early warning indicator
FEFO	first expiry first out
Global Fund	Global Fund to Fight AIDS, Tuberculosis and Malaria
GASP	gonococcal antimicrobial resistance monitoring
GDP	gross domestic product
HIV	human immunodeficiency virus
HMIS	health (management) information system
HOSDID	Hospital Drug Information Database
HSS	HIV sentinel surveillance
IBBS	integrated behavioural and biological surveillance
LPV/r	lopinavir/ritonavir
MDG	Millennium Development Goal
MOH	Ministry of Health
MMM	Mondol Mith Chouy Mith
NATDID	National Drug Information Database
NCHADS	National Center for HIV/AIDS, Dermatology and STDs
NMCHC	National Maternal and Child Health Center
NVP	nevirapine
ODDID	Operational District Drug Information Database
OI	opportunistic infection
PCR	polymerase chain reaction
PDID	Provincial Drug Information Database

PEPFAR		[US] President's Emergency Plan for AIDS Relief
PLHIV		people living with HIV
PMTCT		prevention of mother-to-child transmission [of HIV]
PPP		purchasing power parity
RACHA		Reproductive and Child Health Alliance
RPR		rapid plasma reagin (test for syphilis)
STD		sexually transmitted disease
STI		sexually transmitted infection
TB		tuberculosis
TDF		tenofovir disoproxil fumarate
TPHA		*Treponema pallidum* haemagglutination assay (test for syphilis)
TTI		transfusion-transmitted infection
UNAIDS		Joint United Nations Programme on HIV/AIDS
UNDP		United Nations Development Programme
UNFPA		United Nations Population Fund
UNICEF		United Nations Children's Fund
USAID		United States Agency for International Development
VDRL		Venereal Disease Research Laboratory
WHO		World Health Organization

Introduction

Cambodia faced one of the fastest growing HIV epidemics in Asia in the mid-1990s. Within five years, it became one of the few countries to have reversed the trend. In 2010, Cambodia received a Millennium Development Goal (MDG) award from the United Nations: *"Cambodia is recognized for efforts on HIV that have contributed to a decline in HIV prevalence from an estimated 2% (among adults aged 15–49) in 1998 to 0.8% in 2008. The country has also achieved the universal access target for antiretroviral treatment, with over 90% of adults and children in need receiving treatment."*[1]

The first comprehensive review of the national HIV/AIDS programme of Cambodia was conducted in 1996, followed by periodic evaluations of different thematic areas.[2,3,4,5] The National Center for HIV/AIDS, Dermatology and STDs (NCHADS), Ministry of Health (MOH), requested the World Health Organization (WHO) to support the review of the health sector response to HIV and sexually transmitted infections (STIs).

Purpose and objectives

The initial purpose of the proposed review was to assess the progress made towards the objectives of the Strategic Plan for HIV/AIDS and STI Prevention and Care in Health Sector, 2011–2015. The review focused on the period between 2011 and 2012 with the following objectives:

- assess the progress of the health sector response in terms of coverage, effectiveness, impact and quality of services;
- review the monitoring and evaluation system, including for projects supported by the Global Fund to Fight AIDS, Tuberculosis and Malaria (Global Fund);
- review programme management, interprogramme collaboration, budget allocation and expenditures as well as funding gaps;
- identify gaps and constraints, and areas for further strengthening; and
- provide recommendations for programme planning and management, implementation, and coordination and harmonization among partners.

The review took place at a time when the new conceptual framework for elimination of new HIV infections in Cambodia by 2020 or "Cambodia 3.0" was being finalized. The leadership of NCHADS invited the review team to examine and comment on the contents and feasibility of the new framework and the team agreed to the added objective.

Methods

The review was conducted from 29 April to 10 May 2013 by a team of 23 members consisting of international and local experts, as well as selected staff members of WHO, the Global Fund and national staff, with the support of a local secretariat (Annex I).

Prior to the review, a steering committee was established, consisting of national health staff, members of national and international nongovernmental organizations, representatives of networks of people living with HIV and key populations, and staff of multilateral and bilateral development partners. The steering committee compiled a list of specific issues it wished the review team to explore. Subsequently, the team translated the broad issues figuring on the list into more specific questions relevant to each of the three levels of the national health sector response to HIV, i.e. national, provincial/district and community levels.

The overall scope, schedule and process of the review are outlined in Annex II. The review methods included a desk review, technical briefing by the NCHADS technical teams, interviews with key stakeholders, focused group discussions and observations during site visits in the provinces of Battambang, Banteay Meanchey and Svay Rieng (Annex III), and Phnom Penh (Annex IV).

A pre-review stakeholders meeting (30 April 2013) attended by about 50 participants allowed the review team to introduce the process to partners engaged in HIV work in Cambodia and to receive their insights into specific points of interest needing assessment. The review team then split into several small groups and met with senior officers and staff of NCHADS, National Center for TB and Leprosy Control (CENAT), National Maternal and Child Health Center, National Program of Mental Health, National Institute of Public Health, Department of Planning and Health Information, and Department of Administration and Finance, Department of Administration and Finance of MOH, Ministry of Economy and Finance, Ministry of Interior, University of Health Sciences, the embassies of the United States of America and Australia, and other implementing partners. Altogether, during its visits to Phnom Penh and the three provinces of Battambang, Banteay Meanchey and Svay Rieng, the review team visited three prisons, one detention centre, one drug rehabilitation centre, 20 hospitals and other health facilities (Annex IV). These included four provincial and district hospitals, six health centres and ten community outreach sites. The review team also visited and observed activities at voluntary counselling and testing centres, antenatal clinics, laboratories, blood transfusion centres and pharmaceutical supply stores. The team interviewed 90 health-care workers and counsellors, 23 Mondol Mith Chuoy Mith (MMM) coordinators (network of people living with HIV), 25 community outreach workers, 52 representatives of civil society, and over 100 female and transgender/transsexual entertainment workers, men who have sex with men, people who use drugs including people who inject drugs, managers of entertainment facilities and guest houses, and 45 women and men living with HIV. Overall, around 450 people were interviewed. The assessment team also reviewed close to 450 documents.

The review concluded with the presentation of a short verbal report by the Chair and delegates of the review team to His Excellency Dr Mam Bun Heng, Minister of Health of the Royal Government of Cambodia. It was followed by a stakeholder meeting and validation workshop chaired by His Excellency, the Minister of Health. At this well-attended event, the review team members presented key findings and recommendations. Participants commented on the pertinence, accuracy and completeness of these findings, and pointed out understatements and gaps to which they wished greater attention to be drawn.

In addition to the data collected and compiled during the review, other valuable sources of information were drawn upon. These included, in particular, a preliminary review conducted in January 2013 jointly by the Global Fund and WHO[a] to assess the impact of the response to HIV and identify data needs for future impact assessments; the 2012 report of the review of the Cambodia National Blood Transfusion Services;[6] and the joint TB programme review released in 2013.[7] The recommendations arising from these reports are fully endorsed by this review and several of these will be discussed further in their respective sections. Concerned with the cross-cutting, gender-related determinants of HIV infection and the gender sensitivity of the responses, the review team noted that a gender analysis of the Cambodian health sector had been conducted in 2011,[8] followed by a report on HIV-affected women in Cambodia in 2013.[9] The team was also informed that a further gender analysis, this time focused on the national response to HIV, was planned for the last quarter of 2013.

The 2011 analysis provided a clear assessment and recommendations for strengthening the gender sensitivity and responsiveness of the health sector policies and programmes. Its final report states that *"the assessment of the gender-responsiveness of 12 key policy and strategy documents found the National Reproductive and Maternal and Child Health and the National Strategic Plan for a Comprehensive and Multisectoral Response to HIV/AIDS policies were the most advanced and stood as role models for gender-responsive policy."* The upcoming gender analysis of the response to HIV will create an opportunity to ascertain whether this still holds true in the evolving epidemic context and, as or even more importantly, if the said policies have impacted meaningfully on practices and outcomes. Given these past and upcoming gender analyses, the review team narrowed its own assessment to gender issues related to certain aspects of sexual and reproductive health, gender differentials in access to and use of care and treatment, and in the context of sex work.

Early in July 2013, shortly upon completion of the review, a provisional report was presented, which gave the key findings, conclusions and recommendations.

---

[a] Low-Beer D et al. Impact assessment component of the health sector review of the national HIV programme. January 2013 (unpublished document)

Status and trends of HIV in Cambodia and responses to the epidemics

The history of the emergence of and response to HIV has been marked by an initially intense spread of infection among women and men participating in sex work, followed by an epidemic peak in 1996 and gradual decline ever since. While several factors may have influenced the course of the epidemic, the introduction of the "100% condom use policy" in the late 1990s and the rolling out and rapid scaling up of antiretroviral treatment (ART) from 2005 onwards have been credited with bringing the early epidemic under control and sustaining low rates of HIV transmission. These remarkable results speak of a strong commitment to containing the HIV epidemic, competent and dedicated leadership, and an effective collaboration between the national initiative directed by NCHADS, and international and local nongovernmental organizations and external partners, including development and health agencies and academic entities. The National AIDS Authority (NAA) deserves credit for producing valuable assessment reports on the response to HIV, particularly in 2007, 2010 and 2012, and was about to undertake a further assessment at the time of writing this report.[10] The NAA also plays an active role in the development of policies and formulation of a national comprehensive multisectoral response to HIV/AIDS. This will be referred to in a later section.

Extensive use of modelling methods has been made by NCHADS to estimate and project epidemic and impact trends of HIV in Cambodia.[b] It should be emphasized here that the authors of the report titled *Estimations and projections of HIV/AIDS in Cambodia 2010–2015*[11] have called repeatedly for caution in using the results of this modelling exercise, in view of the extensive array and limitations of numerous assumptions built into the model. Nevertheless, the results of this important modelling exercise have been central to the present report, which cites a number of its findings. According to national estimation and projection models, there were 75 900 adults aged 15 years and above living with HIV in Cambodia in 2010; this figure was projected to decline to 70 400 by 2015, equivalent to a reduction in HIV prevalence from 0.8% in 2010 to 0.7% in 2012, and 0.6% in 2015 (Figure 1).

---

[b] Two models were applied. These models assume that the coverage of the response to HIV/AIDS would remain unchanged till 2015 and any programme or intervention implemented would be comprehensive and of high quality. The model also assumes that the new HIV treatment guidelines for HIV-infected adults (CD4 <350 cells/μL) had been implemented countrywide in 2010, and new treatment guidelines for children (giving ART to those aged less than two years old) had been implemented since 2012. The assumptions and limitations of this modelling exercise are presented on pages 28 and 29 of the report under reference, and its results in subsequent pages.

Figure 1: HIV prevalence among the general population by age groups 15+ and 15–49 years, 1990–2015

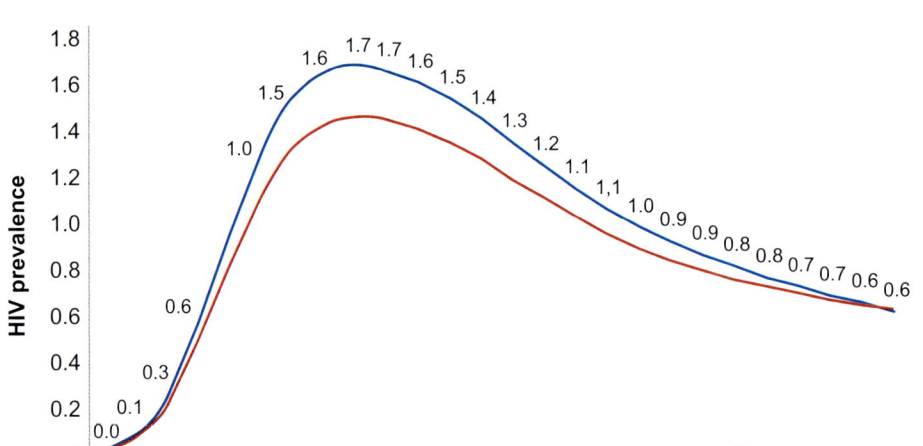

Source: Ministry of Health, National Center for HIV/AIDS, Dermatology and STDs. *Estimations and projections of HIV/AIDS in Cambodia 2010–2015*. Phnom Penh, Cambodia, 2011.

An additional 8512 children aged 0–14 years were estimated to be living with HIV in 2010. This number is also projected to decline to 5497 by 2015 as a result of ageing of this cohort, HIV-related and non-specific mortality, and lower HIV incidence in that age group (Figure 2).[11]

According to the same modelling exercise, HIV-infected women aged 15 years and above accounted for about half of the population of both sexes estimated to be living with HIV in the early 2000s. They are projected to account for about 60% of this population by 2015 (Figure 3). The sex ratio of newly infected individuals aged 15 years and above seems to have stabilized at around that level since 2010. Declining trends in the numbers of newly infected individuals (both sexes combined) aged 15 years and above and women in the same age group have followed similar rates of decline since that time (Figure 4).

Several key populations with high levels of HIV prevalence have been identified (*see* Figure 5). Two recent surveillance studies among female entertainment workers with more than seven clients per week conducted in 2010 (HIV sentinel surveillance [HSS], N=432) and 2011 (STI surveillance survey, N=221) in a large number of provinces (22 and 17, respectively) place the HIV prevalence at 14.0% and 10.0%, respectively. At the 95% confidence interval, these estimates are not statistically distinguishable from one another and are both similar to the previous 2006 prevalence estimate of 14.0% among brothel-based female sex workers.[c,d,12] A surveillance study in 2007 estimated the prevalence at 19–25% among people who inject

---

[c] The change in definition of the study population was made necessary by a new law prohibiting sex work in 2007.

[d] The 95% confidence interval for the 2010 estimate would be approximately 4.5–15.5%, assuming a design effect due to the multistage cluster-sampling design of 2.0, the minimum value typically used for venue-based sampling studies in hidden populations.

Figure 2: Number of HIV-positive children aged 0–14 years and women aged 15 years and above, 2000–2015 (from Spectrum)

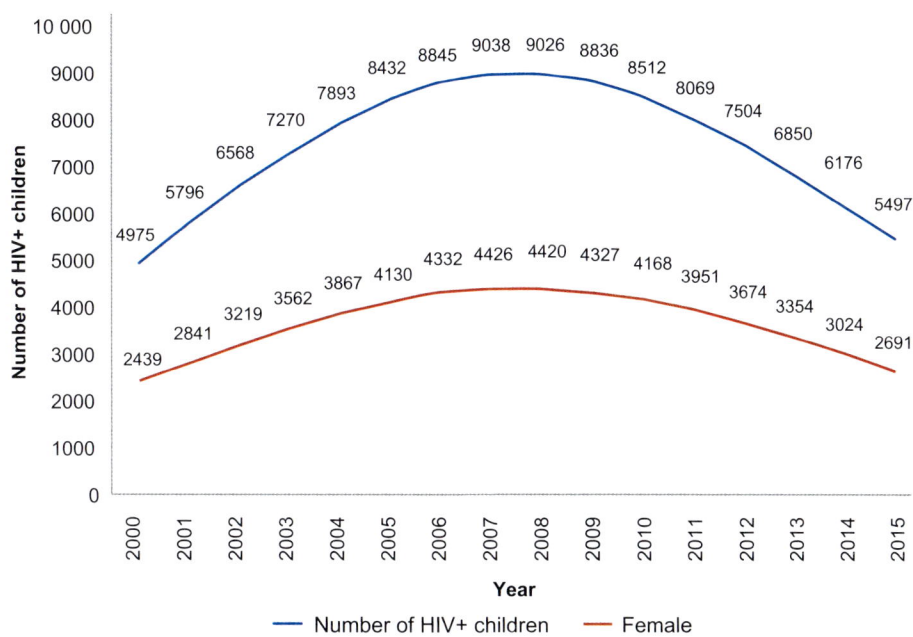

Source: Ministry of Health, National Center for HIV/AIDS, Dermatology and STDs. *Estimations and projections of HIV/AIDS in Cambodia 2010–2015*. Phnom Penh, Cambodia, 2011.

Figure 3: Number of individuals (men and women) and women aged 15 years and above infected with HIV, 1990–2015 (from Spectrum)

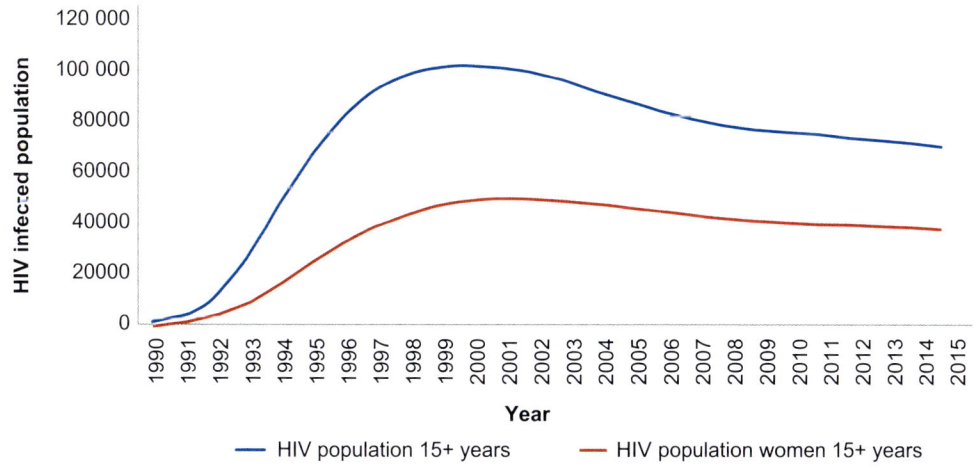

Source: Ministry of Health, National Center for HIV/AIDS Dermatology and STD. *Estimations and projections of HIV/AIDS in Cambodia 2010–2015*. Phnom Penh, Cambodia, 2011.

Figure 4: Number of individuals (men and women) and women aged 15+ years newly infected with HIV, 2000–2015

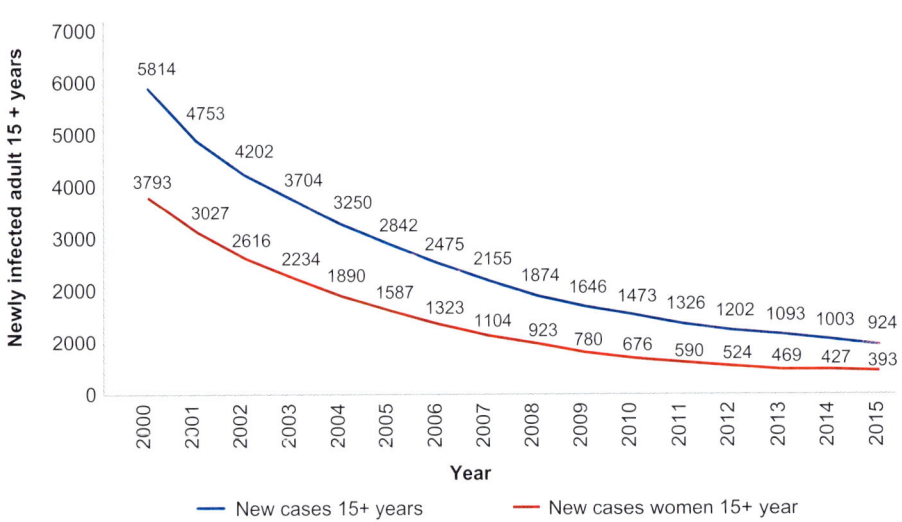

Source: Ministry of Health, National Center for HIV/AIDS, Dermatology and STDs. *Estimations and projections of HIV/AIDS in Cambodia 2010–2015*. Phnom Penh, Cambodia, 2011.

drugs in larger cities, and 0.7–1.3% among non-injecting drug users in 2007.[13] Among men who have sex with men, prevalence was estimated at approximately 2% in 2010; however, an earlier study in 2005 using sampling methods designed for hard-to-reach populations estimated the prevalence at 5% among men who have sex with men overall (9% in Phnom Penh and <1% in two other provinces), and 17% among the subsample of transgender women in Phnom Penh.[14] Ascertaining trends, particularly among sex workers and men who have sex with men, was made difficult by changes in study definitions and methods over time.

Of the 1348 new infections estimated to have occurred in 2012 as shown in Figure 4, almost 50% (678) are estimated to have resulted from heterosexual, non-commercial sexual relationships, about 30% (394) from female sex work, 10% (136) from mother-to-child transmission, less than 10% (125) from injecting drug use, and less than 1% (15) from male-to-male sex.[11] Compared to 2010, new HIV infections from all transmission routes, except through injecting drugs, are expected to have declined, the largest decline being expected for mother-to-child transmission.

The number of individuals in care and treatment has been scaled up rapidly, beginning in 2005. By the end of 2012, 44 318 adults (54% women) and 4595 children (48% girls/young women) were on ART (Table 1), equivalent to a coverage of 81% in adults and 92% in children younger than 14 years of age, respectively (current national guidelines recommend initiation of ART when the CD4 count is below 350 cells/μL).[15] An additional 5204 adults (63% of whom were women) and 1383 children (53% of whom were girls) were active in pre-ART at the end of 2012, equivalent to just 11.9% of all patients in care and treatment. Rates of treatment retention and survival are considerable. Based on three cohorts of individuals initiating ART in 2006, 2009 and 2010, respectively, at approximately half of all ART sites, 93% of patients were still active on ART at 12 months, 84% at 24 months and 78% at 60 months.[16]

Figure 5: HIV prevalence estimates for key-affected populations and pregnant women attending antenatal care from surveillance surveys, 2000–2011

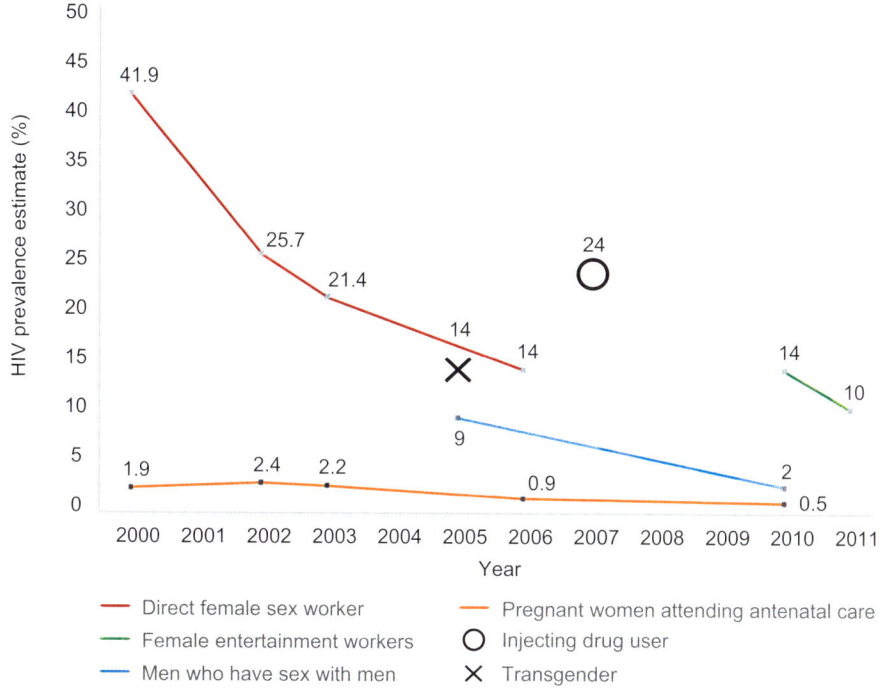

Notes: PP, Phnom Penh (others are national estimates). Surveys among men who have sex with men in 2005 and 2010 used different sampling methods and may not be comparable. Self-identified gender was not considered among the group of men who have sex with men. Transgender (TG) estimate is from a female-identified subsample from the study among men who have sex with men. Confidence intervals are not shown as they are unavailable for most estimates.

The national response to the epidemic

Cambodia was confronted with HIV in extremely vulnerable conditions in the early 1990s as the country was emerging from instability. Fuelled by unprotected sex work, HIV and other STIs spread rapidly through networks of sex workers and clients. Early interventions focusing on HIV and STI prevention in sex work settings began to slow transmission from the mid-1990s, reaching scale with the national roll-out of the 100% condom use programme between 1998 and 2001. Self-reported condom use in sex work increased from less than 40% in 1996 to consistently over 90% between 2001 and 2007 among brothel-based sex workers. More recent estimates among female entertainment workers from the 2010 behavioural surveillance survey (BSS) suggest similar or marginally lower levels of consistent condom use (89% with clients in the past week, 84% in the past three months), which fell to a larger extent in the 2011 STI surveillance survey (76% in the past three months).[e] HIV prevalence among direct brothel-based sex workers decreased from 42% in 1996 to 14% by 2006.[11] Reported STIs declined by more than half between 1996 and 2001 among both sex workers and high-

---

[e] The 2011 condom use estimate is not specific to entertainment workers with more than seven clients, but rather for all female entertainment workers, many of whom had few recent clients and may, therefore, be qualitatively different from brothel-based female sex workers who were the subject of previous surveillance rounds. Similarly, the 2010 estimate is for female entertainment workers with more than two clients on the last working day.

risk males.[17] Considerable scale up of HIV counselling, testing, care and treatment occurred from 2005, possibly offsetting disruptions in other prevention efforts. To be noted is that the treatment coverage rate among people living with HIV was higher in 2009 than in 2012. This apparent decline has to be interpreted against the background of changing criteria for starting ART, from CD4 counts of <200–250 cells/μL in 2009 to CD4 counts <350 cells/μL in 2012.

The responsiveness of the national programme, inclusive of both the formal health sector and civil society, has been a prominent feature of Cambodia's dynamic response to the HIV epidemic. In 2010, Cambodia received an MDG award for outstanding national leadership, commitment and progress towards the achievement of MDG 6, particularly in working towards halting and reversing the spread of HIV. By averting large numbers of "downstream" infections, the early Cambodian response curbed the transmission that was driving the epidemic, later enabling the programme to reach universal access to ART.

Given these coverage trends and their positive impact on survival, the estimated or measured prevalence of HIV in Cambodia (i.e. percentage of the population living with HIV at any point in time) will probably decline more slowly in the coming years as the number of survivors and newly infected women, men and children will offset mortality in the population living with HIV/AIDS, which is estimated to have declined by 77% in the past five years.

HIV transmission from mother to child declined from 25% in 2007 to 11% in 2010, based on national modelling studies. The large increase in antenatal care coverage (from less than 30% in 2005 to over 80% in 2011) has created expectations that the mother-to-child transmission HIV transmission rate can be reduced to below 5%. In 2011, however, more than one third of pregnant women testing positive did not receive antiretroviral (ARV) prophylaxis. The review of the impact of the national response to HIV (January 2013) concluded that to bring the mother-to-child HIV transmission rate to below 5%, Cambodia would need its "boosting strategy" to successfully scale up routine voluntary testing and counselling at points of care and simultaneously provide ART to *all* eligible women. This new approach will require careful evaluation.

As efforts are being deployed to enhance prevention, care and treatment with a particular focus on key-affected populations and women in the reproductive age group, attention has now turned to elimination strategies designed to prevent a constantly shrinking number of new infections. The country has set for itself the ambitious targets outlined in the Cambodia 3.0 framework:[18] (i) to reduce the estimated HIV incidence among the population aged 15 years and older from 18/100 000 in 2010 to 3/100 000 or less by 2020; (ii) to reduce the HIV transmission rate from HIV-positive mothers to their infants from 11–13% in 2010 to 2% or less by 2020; and (iii) to increase the coverage of syphilis screening and treatment to over 95% among pregnant women by 2020.

The Cambodia 3.0 framework encapsulates the key steps to be taken in this direction. It aims at the elimination of new HIV infections through (i) early diagnosis of HIV infection, and early access to ART as prevention and a boosted continuum of care, (ii) boosted prev ention of mother-to-child HIV transmission, (iii) boosted access to and utilization of prevention, care and treatment services by key-affected populations, (iv) strengthening of community-based health services, and (v) enhanced monitoring and evaluation of impacts.

Table 1. Antiretroviral treatment coverage as of 2012 [11, 58]

	(a) Estimated number of PLHIV in Cambodia, 2012	(b) Estimated number eligible for ART	(c) Estimated % of PLHIV eligible ART in 2012 (c=e/b)	(d) Ratio PLHIV M/W eligible for ART	(e) Reported number of PLHIV on ART	(f) Estimated % of PLHIV receiving ART (f=e/a)	(g) Ratio M/W PLHIV on ART
Adults 15+ years	74 572 (100%)	55 036 (100%)	81%	0.88	44 318 (100%)	59%	0.85
Women	40 179 (54%)	29 269 (54%)	82%		23 932 (54%)	60%	
Men	34 993 (46%)	25 767 (46%)	79%		20 386 (46%)	58%	
Children <15 years	7 504 (100%)	4 997 (100%)	92%	1.04	4 595 (100%)	61%	1.08
Girls	3 674 (49%)	2 448 (49%)	90%		2 205 (48%)		
Boys	3 830 (51%)	2 549 (51%)	94%		2 390 (52%)		

(a) Total estimated number of PLHIV through modelling (Percentage indicates the proportion of females and males in adults and children, respectively.) (Adapted from Chhorvann et al. 2011. Estimations and projections of HIV/AIDS in Cambodia 2010–2015, figures 29 and 33).[11]
(b) Estimated through modelling (Percentage indicates proportion of females and males in adults and children, respectively.) (Adapted from Chhorvann et al. 2011. Estimations and projections of HIV/AIDS in Cambodia 2010–2015, figures 31 and 35).[11]
(c) Estimated percentage of estimated PLHIV eligible for receiving ART in 2012.
(d) Gender ratio of men/women eligible for ART in 2012 (estimated).
(e) Reported number of PLHIV on ART (Percentage indicates the proportion of females and males in adults and children, respectively.).
(f) Estimated percentage of PLHIV receiving ART.
(g) Gender ratio (M/W) of eligible PLHIV receiving ART (reported).

Findings and recommendations

A summary of the findings and recommendations of the review is given below. This document does not cover exhaustively all facets of the HIV situation in Cambodia and of the responses brought against it. The scope of the review was limited because of the vast array of issues pertaining to HIV in the country, such as preponderance of certain issues over others, limited availability of readily accessible and appropriate data, and specificity of evaluation methods required to probe into certain epidemiological, technical or operational questions. Accordingly, the review team devoted most of its resources, time and attention to such programmatic areas as policies and governance; strategic information; continuum of prevention, care and treatment in programme delivery, particularly for key-affected populations; procurement of medicines and biomedical supplies; and financing. Themes that are not extensively addressed in this report but considered under several broader topics include the following: community response and home-based care; paediatric and adolescent HIV prevention, treatment, care and support services; functional linkages between HIV, hepatitis B and C, and noncommunicable diseases; the interplay between HIV and health systems strengthening; interaction between NCHADS and civil society; and mobility among key-affected populations.

1. Policy, strategy and structures

The national multisectoral response to HIV operates under the purview of the NAA, a leading and coordinating entity established in 1999. The NAA reports to the Prime Minister who has delegated this responsibility to the Deputy Prime Minister. The NAA is mandated to foster and monitor coordination on HIV/AIDS matters across 29 government ministries and 24 provinces, and is also tasked with mobilizing resources in support of the multisectoral response to HIV/AIDS. In practice, it operates within the scope of the Strategic Plan for HIV/AIDS and STI Prevention and Care in Health Sector, 2011–2015 for Cambodia, for which aid effectiveness is coordinated through a panel of 19 government–donor joint technical working groups, bringing together national representatives of a particular sector and representatives of civil society, and bilateral and multilateral development agencies. The NAA chairs and is responsible for the effective functioning of the government–donor joint technical working group on HIV/AIDS. NCHADS is a member of two of these technical working groups, one on health and the other on HIV/AIDS. The NAA has an important leading and consultative role in sectoral policy development on HIV/AIDS-related matters, although its advice is not always sought. To illustrate this point, the Ministry of Interior did not solicit the NAA's views when it was developing policies on human trafficking, safe communities or combating drugs. A mid-term review of progress achieved under the multisectoral National Strategic Plan for Comprehensive and Multisectoral Response to HIV/AIDS III (2011–2015) will be carried out in 2013 across key sectors directly concerned with HIV/AIDS. The health sector's response to HIV will not be part of that review as it was reviewed separately and in some depth in May 2013 (the present report), but it is hoped that both processes will at some point converge so as to determine optimal ways to ensure a reinforced, bidirectional relationship between the NAA and NCHADS.

For all purposes, NCHADS operates as the executive branch of the MOH charged with the responsibility of guiding, implementing, monitoring, evaluating and raising resources in support of the health sector response to HIV and STIs (Figure 6). This includes biological and behavioural surveillance and surveys. To this end, it has, over the years, developed and nurtured active collaboration with diverse partners and implementing agencies, both within the formal health sector and nongovernmental organizations. It has a strong leadership, a robust staff at its central office, a streamlined chain of technical guidance and support, supervision, strategic information flow and analysis, and financing extending to the provinces, operational districts and health centres. When necessary, it has the capacity for engaging jointly with other ministries, as is the case with the Ministry of Interior for HIV in prisons.

NCHADS's reputation as a dynamic and successful entity extends beyond the boundaries of the nation. It is credited with having spearheaded one of the most creative and successful responses to HIV in low-/medium-income countries. Its vision and actions are currently guided by: (i) a multisectoral strategic plan on HIV/AIDS, 2011–2015, developed under the auspices of the NAA; and (ii) a Strategic Plan for HIV/AIDS and STI Prevention and Care in the Health Sector,[20] developed by NCHADS and the MOH and complemented by annual action plans produced at the central and provincial levels. Typically, NCHADS updates its strategies periodically based on experience, shifting needs and priorities, the emergence of new technologies and international best practices. These updates, which introduce new interventions often intended to boost the implementation of specific elements of the strategy, are translated into an

Figure 6: Structure and organization of the Ministry of Health

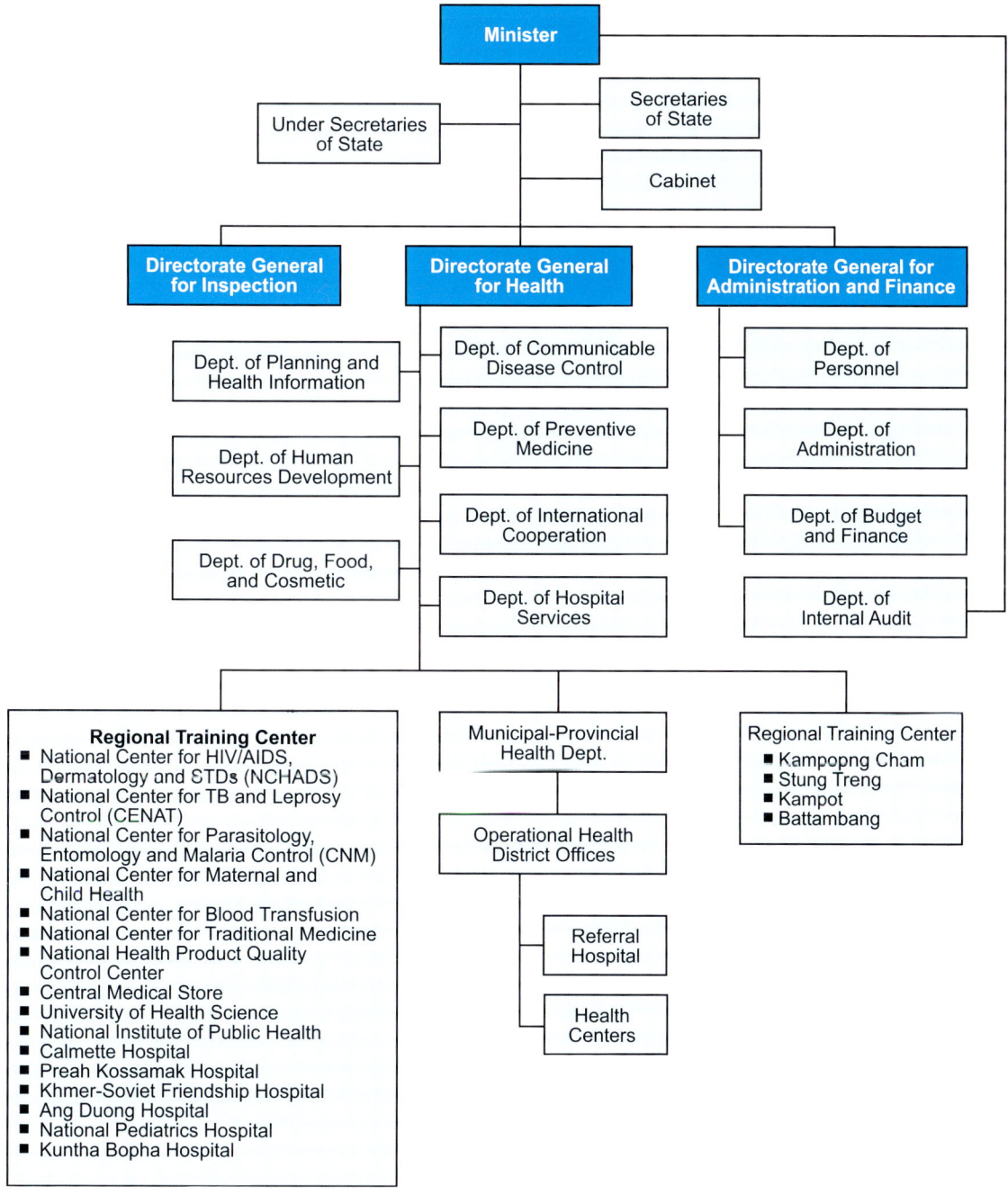

ever-growing number of standard operating procedures and concept notes, each bringing in its trail additional needs for training, financing and monitoring. While these periodic changes contribute to improvement of programme outcomes, the flurry of standard operating procedures and other guidance documents to be followed by central and peripheral staff add their own burden to an already overloaded and complex assembly of technical and operational documents. Recognizing this state of affairs, the new strategy currently being finalized, Cambodia 3.0, will aim at consolidating strategic approaches and the documentation supporting them.

The health sector has made considerable strides in responding vigorously to the HIV epidemic, prevented many new infections and provided thousands of women, men and children living with HIV with the prospect of a longer and better quality of life. HIV is now considered as a chronic condition. This response must be further enhanced, adapted to the evolving nature of the epidemic of HIV infection and the global economic landscape, and sustained in the long term. In its effort to enhance synergies within the health sector by strengthening linkages between its departments and initiatives, the MOH must now determine how and along what time line the health sector response to HIV will gradually be aligned with other health sector priorities in a mutually supportive fashion. Such a change in strategy could consider key factors that will ensure that it catalyses synergies and avoids impeding further progress in the national response to HIV (*see* Box 1). It seems important to the review team to preserve and continue to strengthen the structure and the technical and operational capacity of NCHADS until a comprehensive roadmap for alignment within the MOH is successfully completed, a process that is likely to require a minimum of two years.

With a typical staff shortage of around 10% in peripheral health facilities, the health sector response to HIV and STIs suffers from inadequate recruitment, training and employment of skilled staff. The staff turnover and resulting loss of skilled personnel are high and growing as health professionals move away from government services to more attractive private or international employments. A large and growing proportion of human resources for health operate under time-limited contracts. Related to these trends is the fact that the income of government health sector personnel contributing to the response to HIV and STIs is highly inadequate to ensure their sustained dedication to this constantly expanding effort, their responsiveness to growing demands for their services, and the appropriate use of resources made available to them. The suspension of the incentive scheme in January 2013 has been the source of much dissatisfaction and loss of morale across the entire staff, leading many of them to lower their level of performance as they had to search for alternate sources of income for economic survival.

In 2012, total spending on HIV was estimated at around US$ 51 million, of which 11% in 2012 was contributed by domestic public funding. Other resources came from external donors, in particular the Global Fund, which covered 45% of the international funding, the rest being mainly provided by the US government (United States Agency for International Development [USAID], Centers for Disease Control

---

Box 1. Goals of the proposed changes in strategy for the health sector response to HIV and STI

(1) To maintain the leadership of NCHADS in implementing responses to HIV and STIs, and adapting these to evolving epidemiological realities and service needs;

(2) To devolve greater authority and resources to provinces and operational districts, along with strengthened capacity for planning, implementation and accountability at these levels;

(3) To achieve greater collaboration between and encourage appropriate use of resources across departments and initiatives of the health sector engaged in the response to HIV and STI, in particular, those concerned with tuberculosis, maternal and child health, and primary health care, noncommunicable diseases, mental health, health systems strengthening and strategic information systems;

(4) To consolidate relationships with civil society on the basis of judicious sharing of responsibilities and resources, and mutual accountability on health-related matters, and explore collaborative opportunities with the private health sector, using HIV as an entry point; and

(5) To move towards greater harmony in resource mobilization and financing mechanisms within the health sector.

and Prevention [CDC]), with contributions from other bilateral donors, the United Nations system and international nongovernmental organizations. The extreme reliance of the Cambodian health sector response to HIV/AIDS on external funding sources and the prominence of a single funding source over all donors to the programme does not bode well for its long-term sustainability or the risk of abrupt and unanticipated discontinuation of funding.

While recommendations for improving the scope and quality of services within the health sector response to HIV and STIs will appear under different sections of the review findings, below are a few recommendations on key policy, structural, functional and human resource aspects of this response.

Recommendations

1.1 The alignment about to begin within the MOH departments and initiatives may be arranged in a way that generates synergies, with expanded benefits accruing to all concerned programmes, while protecting and nurturing their respective gains.

1.2 During 2013–2014, it is suggested that a feasibility assessment be carried out and a roadmap drawn to further adapt the role and functions of NCHADS to (i) the evolving HIV/STI situation, (ii) the strategic changes reflected in the new conceptual framework, and (iii) the health sector capacity in the country. Till the assessment is done, it would be best to preserve the structure, management and staff of NCHADS at the present level.

1.3 By actively pursuing the development of operational plans of the Cambodia 3.0 framework, NCHADS would be taking advantage of the opportunity to remedy the fragmentation of programme strategies resulting from an ever-expanding series of interventions. Interventions, related standard operating procedures and performance monitoring could be consolidated in the form of a compact, outcome-driven programme informed by evidence.

1.4 By the end of 2014, the MOH would have developed its change strategy in consultation with other partners within the health sector and funding agencies. The MOH could then engage with determination in a transition towards more effective linkages on HIV across concerned departments and initiatives within the health sector and with external partners. While NCHADS would remain the backbone of the national response to HIV and STIs in the near future, it is important that it play a central role in the elaboration and unfolding of the change strategy in its domain of activity (*see* Box 1).

1.5 Given the alarming trends in staff shortages and turnover, there is an urgent need to reinforce the human resources capacity in the formal health sector. The recently produced definition of roles and tasks of NCHADS is an important step in this direction. The review team recommends that, within the MOH, the Department of Human Resources under the Directorate General for Health and the Department of Personnel under the Directorate of Administration and Finance jointly formulate a plan to respond to this pressing issue.

1.6 The salary scale and associated incentives offered to the health workforce should match the current economic reality in Cambodia, and ensure that the retention and good performance of the human resources engaged in combating HIV/STI are valued and protected. The review team urges the Minister of Health, the Council of Administrative Reform and higher authorities to deal with this matter urgently. Failing to do so may lead to further degradation of the livelihood and morale of health staff, and impede the performance of the system.

1.7 Strengthening the interaction between the NAA and NCHADS would be beneficial. The review team took note of the upcoming mid-term review of the multisectoral strategic plan on HIV undertaken by the NAA. In order to avoid duplication of efforts, this review agreed not to cover the health sector. The review team recommends that the outcome of the present health sector's response to HIV be considered in the broader multisectoral review, and that, in return, the findings of the review of the multisectoral response to HIV inform the health sector's response to HIV so as to create mutually beneficial synergies.

1.8 It is suggested that the MOH, through NCHADS, ensure that the recommendations contained in this report are translated into an operational plan, implemented with the needed support and followed up.

2. Creating an enabling environment

Assessing and adjusting harmful policies and laws

As Cambodia's HIV epidemic shifted from a generalized to a more concentrated pattern, increasingly focused on key populations at highest risk, the importance of an enabling environment to optimize the effectiveness of interventions with these populations became even more critical.[21] On the 2020 horizon, the rapid decline in HIV incidence, expected soon to dip below 1000 new infections per year, means that newly infected individuals are and will be increasingly difficult to find. Over time, broad-based case-finding efforts will yield diminishing returns, while it will be increasingly important to detect and interrupt ongoing HIV transmission within high-risk networks. Reaching hidden pockets of marginal and highly vulnerable individuals with effective interventions requires an environment where trust can be established, peer interventions can operate openly and needed services of optimal quality can be accessed.

The elimination of new infections also requires retention within an effective continuum of HIV prevention, care and treatment – from awareness-raising and education on HIV transmission to prevention, including behaviour change, to diagnosis of HIV infection, referral of HIV-positive individuals for pre-ART and ART, and sustained adherence to therapy supported by clinical and biological monitoring. Reducing the rates of drop-out and loss to follow up at each of these steps also depends on creating and maintaining an enabling environment.

Case-finding has a critical role to play in ensuring the early detection of people living with HIV, while epidemiological and behavioural surveillance informs the programme of ongoing and newly emerging trends of HIV and associated infections, risk-taking behaviours and societal vulnerability. An enabling environment is crucial to the success of such efforts. Both discrimination against those infected or affected by HIV and adverse laws and policies can create a climate of fear among key-affected populations who, as a result, move "underground", avoiding surveys as well as needed health and social services (*see* Box 2).

Box 2. Eradicating HIV-related discrimination

Although many key informants, in particular among the health staff, stated that stigma and discrimination associated with HIV had declined considerably in Cambodia over the past decade, the review team received accounts of active discrimination perpetrated against people living with HIV, particularly within the health sector. These concerned women in particular, especially in the context of sexual and reproductive health services. Women living with HIV who were interviewed reported that they were reluctantly attended to by health staff, or even denied basic services, and often not informed about their reproductive choices. These women avoided attending health services because of the fear of poor treatment. This state of affairs must change in accordance with human rights standards and the 2002 Cambodian "HIV law" which stipulates (Article 41): "Discrimination against person with HIV/AIDS in the hospitals and health institutions is strictly prohibited."[f,22]

A network of HIV-positive women reported to the review team

"In general, women don't seek treatment until sick. Doctor provides prescription but patient cannot ask questions. At the health facility, they gather all women living with HIV separately from non-infected women. It is hard for people living with HIV to access surgical services. Surgeon may recommend an operation but delays the operation when the HIV-positive status of the patient is discovered. There are many other examples of discrimination in the health-care environment."

See also *People living with HIV stigma index study in Cambodia: the quantitative findings*. Presented by Ung Mengieng, Research Associate, Strategic Information Department, KHANA. Available at:

http://www.phnompenhsymposium.org/doc/TRACKB/B10_People%20Living%20with%20HIV%20Stigma%20Index%20Study.pdf

---

[f] The Law on the Prevention and Control of HIV/AIDS was enacted by the National Assembly on 14 June 2002 at its eighth plenary session of the second legislature, and its form and legal concepts entirely approved by the Senate on 10 July 2002 at its seventh plenary session of the first legislature.

Since 2007, the enactment of a new addition to the laws on suppression of human trafficking and sexual exploitation was followed by a nationwide crackdown on brothels and police sweeps of outdoor-based sex workers.[23,24] Part of the sex worker population (renamed entertainment workers) moved to establishments such as massage parlours, beer gardens and karaoke bars where contacts between entertainment workers and prospective clients could be made.[g,25] Following such contacts, sexual encounters may occur in neighbouring "guesthouses". Peer educators and health staff engaged in HIV work such as prevention, including condom distribution, promotion of HIV testing, treatment of STIs and referral, now reach this population relatively easily. But there are other women (and male and transgender sex workers) who do not use entertainment venues or who contact prospective clients independently. Implementation of this new law makes access to these hidden populations problematic. In November 2008, responding to pressure from sex worker groups supported by HIV/AIDS health and social workers and civil society groups, and to avoid inappropriate interpretations of the law by law enforcement officials or the judicial system, the High-level Inter-agency Anti-Trafficking Task Force issued the Guidelines on Implementation of the Law on Trafficking and Sexual Exploitation.[26] These guidelines and an explanatory note issued shortly thereafter were intended to reduce harmful interpretations of the law. Officials of the Ministry of Interior acknowledged during the review that they were aware of the adverse consequences of the law on the ability of sex workers to protect themselves and their clients against HIV. They stated that, to their knowledge, the situation had improved but that much remained to be done to disseminate and promote the guidelines and explanatory note among law enforcement officers and concerned social protection institutions.

Through an interministerial technical working group, the Ministry of Interior had developed enabling policies for harm reduction in Phnom Penh in the early 2000s. Over the ensuing decade, two nongovernmental organizations developed outreach distribution programmes for clean injecting equipment in the capital, while methadone treatment was offered by the MOH. In 2010, however, the Ministry of Interior launched the Village/Commune Safety policy.[27] The policy urged authorities at the commune level to ensure that there was no stealing, drug production or dealing, prostitution, child trafficking, domestic violence, gangsters, illegal gaming, and use of illegal weapons or crime occurring in any commune in Cambodia. (This list was extended from five original components to nine.) If reports or evidence indicated that a person distributed drugs, this person would be arrested and prosecuted. The fear created by this law and its interpretation by local law enforcement officers resulted in drug-using populations being reluctant to identify themselves to outreach health services, reducing needle and syringe distribution by one nongovernmental organization by a factor of three and being associated with an increase in loss to follow up for those on methadone. It should be noted that during the review, the National Authority for Combating Drugs indicated to reviewers that individuals carrying small amounts of drugs for personal consumption would not be arrested, though there remains substantial fear among these very high-risk populations.

Beyond the legal framework, promotion of a dialogue for changing social norms plays a critical role in creating a more enabling environment and improving the uptake of health services, especially at the local and community levels. Considerable efforts have been made over the past few years to mitigate the negative impacts of the existing legislations. The review team found that the provincial law enforcement authorities are increasingly recognizing the need for such efforts and that they plan to expand their efforts over the next few years. To facilitate this process, increased collaboration with law enforcement institutions is explicitly included in the Conceptual Framework of Cambodia 3.0, in particular, with regard to the continuum of prevention, care and treatment for key populations at greatest risk. It is also important to mention that the standard operating procedure for implementing the Boosted Continuum of Prevention to Care and Treatment for key-affected populations includes a Police–Community Partnership Initiative with the aim of ensuring a safe and enabling environment for these populations.[h]

---

[g] This reference gives a detailed description and analysis of structures, patterns and context of sex work in Cambodia.

[h] Continuum Prevention to Care and Treatment (CoPCT), draft 25, Section 10: enabling environment (focusing on the roles of police). NCHADS, Ministry of Health (unpublished document).

Recommendations

2.1 The creation of an enabling environment for the response to HIV requires that the benefits and risks associated with every policy enacted by any branch of the government be assessed from a dual HIV and public security perspective before being promulgated. The method of health impact assessment could be used to project the possible impact of proposed new policies and laws on HIV. This method is increasingly being applied in the South-East Asia and Western Pacific regions (*see* Box 3).

2.2 Implementation of existing and planned initiatives such as the Police–Community Partnership Initiative designed to strengthen enabling environments should receive high priority under the Boosted Continuum of Prevention to Care and Treatment, and be adequately monitored and periodically assessed against their intended outcomes.

2.3 The MOH should make the health workforce more familiar with the 2002 HIV law. It is important to retrain health staff in providing services and being responsive to the special needs of men, women and children living with HIV. It would also be helpful to provide opportunities for health workers to express their fears rationally and fulfil their obligations professionally through group discussions in which peers and people living with HIV should participate.

Box 3. Health impact assessment

"Health impact assessment (HIA) is a practical approach to judge the potential health effects of a policy, programme or project on a population, particularly on vulnerable or disadvantaged groups. Recommendations are produced by decision-makers and stakeholders, with the aim of maximizing the proposal's positive health effects and minimizing its negative health effects. [...]

"Health impact assessment provides a way to engage with members of the public affected by a particular proposal. A health impact assessment can send a signal that an organization or partnership wants to involve a community and is willing to respond constructively to their concerns. Because the assessment process values many different types of evidence, the views of the public can be considered alongside expert opinion and scientific data, with each source of information being valued equally. It is important to note that the decision-makers may value certain types of evidence more than others and community expectations must be managed to avoid over-promising what that assessment can deliver. A health impact assessment does not make decisions; it provides information in a clear and transparent way for decision-makers."

Excerpts from *Health impact assessment: why use HIA?* Geneva; World Health Organization. Available at: http://www.who.int/hia/about/why/en/index1.html (accessed 29 April 2014).

---

3. Strategic information

Cambodia's HIV epidemic has evolved dramatically over the past decade, with declines in HIV prevalence from 2.2% in 2003 to 0.5% in 2010 among pregnant women.[28] HIV prevalence has also declined among women engaged in commercial sex, from a peak of 45.8% among brothel-based sex workers in 1998 to 21.4% in 2003, to 10–14.0% in 2010 among entertainment workers with more than seven clients per week.[29] New populations at increased risk have also been identified in this period, specifically people who inject drugs,[29,30] transgender women and men who have sex with men.[17] Surveillance has been essential to identifying changes over the course of the epidemic to date, providing supporting evidence of the effectiveness of interventions and of increased prevalence levels in risk groups. As the epidemic continues to evolve, and as the country intensifies its rapid scale-up of HIV testing, treatment, outreach and prevention under the Cambodia 3.0 strategy, surveillance and programme monitoring will continue to be critical to assess changes and progress in a timely manner, so that programmes can be adjusted accordingly. Scale up will bring new challenges in maintaining and improving programme quality, making monitoring even more important. Similarly, reaching targets for reducing the incidence of infections is likely to become more difficult as the incidence declines.

This review examined four topics related to strategic information at the request of the steering committee: surveillance, mapping and population size estimates for populations most at risk, quality improvement systems, and monitoring linkages across the services cascade.

Surveillance: keeping pace with an evolving epidemic

Surveillance studies

Biological surveillance studies to assess the prevalence of HIV infection have consistently provided a robust picture of the national epidemic, with studies conducted since the mid-1990s among pregnant women and female entertainment workers and, more recently, among men who have sex with men and people who use drugs (this includes injecting drug users as well as those who smoke and take oral drugs). Studies to assess the prevalence of other STIs have been conducted among entertainment workers since 2001[31,32] and among men who have sex with men in 2005 and 2010.[17,33]

Behavioural surveys to characterize risk and access to services have been conducted in parallel and are being integrated with biological surveillance in recent times. Together, these studies have provided the data needed for epidemic models, which are routinely used to estimate and project national trends in HIV prevalence, incidence and mortality.

In addition to developing national estimates, data from surveillance studies can be invaluable for discerning local epidemic trends. This will become more important as Cambodia 3.0's goal of eliminating all new infections increasingly moves the country toward finer targeting of prevention efforts (*see* Section 4). HIV prevalence among antenatal women continues to exceed 1.0% in some provinces, pointing to an uneven distribution of the HIV burden.[28] The review team also heard from local health departments that the source of new infections and the relative importance of risk groups locally are often not well understood. Differences in epidemic burden across Cambodia's 24 provinces could be due to a number of factors, including varying degrees of urbanization and population density; differences in HIV knowledge and patterns of risk behaviours; the size of risk groups; contextual factors such as borders with neighbouring Thailand, Viet Nam and the Lao People's Democratic Republic, and patterns of in- and out-migration; and varying levels of prevention strategies or responsiveness to these factor. Data from surveillance studies and programmatic data could both be leveraged to improve understanding of the local drivers of HIV transmission. While antenatal sentinel surveillance studies rely on robust provincial samples (400 participants per province in 2010, enough to estimate a prevalence of 1% with an error of about 1%), samples of risk groups surveyed outside of Phnom Penh have been smaller (186 sex workers per province in the 2010 HSS and 124 to 100 men who have sex with men per province in 2005 and 2010, respectively). Given the greater chances of error associated with the sampling methods used to reach these populations (venue-based sampling for sex workers, respondent-driven sampling for men who have sex with men), a sample size of 300 or more is generally recommended to produce informative estimates at each study site. This would most likely be feasible in Cambodia's larger cities, such as Battambang and Siem Reap. However, formative research ahead of future studies could help to determine where increasing the sample size would be feasible.

NCHADS has demonstrated its ability to adopt new surveillance methods when needed. For example, the 2005 study among men who have sex with men and the recent 2012 study among people who inject drugs used sampling methods designed specifically for hard-to-reach populations. Yet, there is concern that higher-risk subgroups of sex workers, men who have sex with men and people who inject drugs may not be adequately reflected in surveillance data. This suggests that a review is needed of study recruitment strategies and their implementation in practice.

Surveillance studies in risk groups can also contribute to monitoring the levels of transmitted resistance of HIV to antiretroviral medications. As the incidence of HIV declines fewer HIV cases will be detected through routine testing programmes. Incorporating transmitted drug resistance surveys in surveillance studies conducted among risk groups with a high HIV prevalence, as has been done elsewhere,[34] may help to address this gap.

Finally, NCHADS has achieved very high levels of coverage of HIV testing in antenatal settings. Estimates of HIV prevalence based on routine testing data are therefore increasingly representative of the antenatal population. In this circumstance, surveillance studies using unlinked anonymous testing may no longer be needed to provide unbiased prevalence estimates among antenatal women. NCHADS and partners are preparing to conduct a comparison of these sources of data and should consider relying exclusively on programme data if findings indicate close agreement with survey data at the facility, province and national levels.

HIV case reporting

HIV case reporting is based on test results from 253 voluntary counselling and testing centres located at government hospitals and health clinics, and nongovernmental organizations. Individuals seeking testing are largely walk-ins and referrals from antenatal clinics (84% in 2011), as well as referrals from specialized STI clinics, tuberculosis (TB) and other health services, primarily from public sector health facilities. While an individual-level database containing test results and a standardized behavioural assessment is in place at a limited number of voluntary counselling and testing centres, HIV reports prepared at the facility level are aggregated by age, sex and source of referral, and then aggregated further by operational districts,[i] provincial health departments and NCHADS. Facilities prepare the aggregated count data by using the electronic database or manually from facility registers, particularly at sites where no working computer is available. A similar system is in place for syndromic and etiological reporting of STIs.

The HIV reporting system currently does not include routine procedures to detect and eliminate double-counting of individuals who have presented for testing previously, whether at the same facility or at different facilities. Repeat testers who are positive will lead to overestimation of the number of new HIV cases and the percentage of individuals who test positive. Repeat testers who are negative will lead to underestimation of positivity among individuals tested. Data describing repeat HIV testers are not available to determine the net effect of double-counting on reporting results. The current design of the patient monitoring systems also makes it difficult to capture information on partners or couples tested, and does not link partners and couples to allow for analysis of the percentage of partners tested, among other outcomes.[35,36]

National voluntary counselling and testing reports prepared by the NCHADS data management unit do not present trends, but they do present the number of HIV tests, their results, their demographic characteristics and source of referral categories. The use of these data could be greatly improved by characterizing trends among individuals who test positive, by adding data from behavioural assessments. This information would facilitate understanding of the association of trends with risk factors. Currently, this information is available only through mathematical modelling.

Assessing HIV incidence

Detecting changes in HIV incidence – the rate at which new infections are acquired – is important for two reasons: (i) to measure progress towards Cambodia 3.0's goals to eliminate new HIV infections, and (ii) to direct prevention to subgroups and areas where transmission is greatest.

In Cambodia, HIV incidence was estimated for sex workers and antenatal women using laboratory assays as recently as 2006,[j] but has not been included in more recent surveillance studies,[37] most likely due to a global debate regarding the technical limitations of available incidence assays. As new assays have become available, recent guidance from WHO and the Joint United Nations Programme on HIV/AIDS (UNAIDS) recommends that countries continue to incorporate incidence testing in surveillance studies.[38] At present, incidence estimates are available only through models.

---

[i] In 1995, the Ministry of Health approved a new health system that aimed at improving and extending primary health care through "District-based health system", also known as operational district. As of 2006, there were eight national hospitals, 77 operational districts, 69 referral hospitals and 972 health centres and 79 health posts.

[j] NCHADS Surveillance Unit. HIV sentinel surveillance 2006. Powerpoint presentation, 15 August 2008

Data from sentinel surveillance in Cambodia could support a second method to track incidence; namely, examining changes over time in HIV prevalence among young antenatal women (i.e. under 24 years, or 20 years if the data allow). Reports to date have not presented this kind of trend analysis. In addition to data from antenatal studies, analysis of trends from routine HIV testing of young antenatal women provides an additional source of evidence regarding changes in incidence. Given the importance of assessing the impact of prevention strategies and monitoring progress toward HIV elimination, it would be desirable to triangulate the incidence estimates from national epidemic models with these additional data sources.

Recommendations

3.1 It is recommended that strategies by which surveillance studies in risk groups could be strengthened to improve upon city-/provincial-level estimates, especially for larger cities and those areas with the greatest epidemic burden, be assessed by a national working group on HIV strategic information. Evaluating different options would help to ensure that the most critical information is collected at minimal cost.

3.2 It is recommended that trend analysis of the sociodemographic and behavioural characteristics of individuals who test positive for HIV at voluntary counselling and testing sites be included in their programme reports. It needs to be explored whether such trends can best be ascertained by analysis of individual-level databases or by introducing HIV case reporting (i.e. individual-level instead of aggregate-level reporting) with confidentiality protections. Given the likelihood of underreporting of stigmatized risk behaviours, data from voluntary counselling and testing sites should be triangulated with other data sources, such as data from outreach programmes and surveillance studies.

3.3 Current efforts are warranted by NCHADS and partners to assess the feasibility of using routine data from prevention of mother-to-child transmission (PMTCT) programmes instead of unlinked, anonymous HIV testing for surveillance purposes. Issues to be explored include the level of agreement of prevalence estimates between data from routine PMTCT services and unlinked, anonymous HIV testing at antenatal clinic facilities; the impact of selection bias on prevalence estimates using PMTCT programme data; and the potential impact of using service-based data for surveillance purposes on attendance at antenatal clinic services.

3.4 It is recommended that analyses be developed to assess trends in HIV incidence based on trends in prevalence among young antenatal attendees <24 years (or <20 years if the data allow) and incidence trends determined in integrated biological and behavioural surveillance (IBBS) studies by newly developed assays.

Mapping and estimating the size of key-affected populations

The HIV programme and nongovernmental organizations conduct regular mapping exercises to estimate the number of entertainment workers and men who have sex with men in local areas, which are then aggregated to the national level. These estimates provide the data needed to produce national estimates and projections of the epidemic. Importantly, size estimates provide denominators for key indicators such as outreach coverage and utilization of health services by key populations. They are therefore essential to both high-level analysis of epidemic trends and implementation of prevention programmes. Moreover, accurate mapping is essential for better targeting of the highest-risk populations (see Section 4).

The methods used by nongovernmental organizations throughout the country to map risk groups vary widely and thus do not lend themselves to cross-site comparisons. There is also concern that the methods in use may not adequately cover populations potentially at higher risk, such as street-based sex workers and more hidden injection drug users and men who have sex with men. Recognizing this, NCHADS and nongovernmental organizations are examining internationally recognized methodologies to improve the quality and uniformity of mapping and mapping-based size estimates. While mapping is critical for targeting prevention activities, size estimates based on mapping are problematic for risk populations: they may double-count those who frequent venues most and miss those who frequent venues least. Recent surveillance surveys in men who have sex with men and people who use drugs have incorporated methods that are more appropriate for hidden populations, such as the multiplier method.[39,40]

However, because estimation error is large when using the multiplier methods and other size estimation methods, several estimates should be developed: there is greater confidence when several estimates point to a similar result. NCHADS can attain several size estimates from surveillance studies in the future by drawing on its myriad programmatic databases—from outreach to voluntary counselling and testing to treatment. However, this will require a sustained effort to standardize how utilization of services by risk populations is measured by each service. Additionally, the current efforts to introduce a unique identifier to eliminate duplication across services and programmes will be critical to ensure the quality of the multiplier estimates. Careful planning will be necessary well ahead of future studies to ensure that compatible data from various services are ready when they are required.

Recommendations

3.5 It is suggested that current efforts continue by NCHADS and partners to standardize methods for mapping and size estimation of key-affected populations. A national plan is recommended to ensure that estimates are reliable and updated regularly (every two years). The plan would need to define methods for both mapping (as a part of routine programme management) and population size estimation (derived from mapping and surveillance surveys) for the population in each city/province, with standard definitions and timelines. It is recommended that efforts to strengthen programmatic data quality and use these in conjunction with surveys to develop the size estimates be included in the plan. As improved methods become available (every three to four years), it is suggested that the existing methods be reviewed and revised.

3.6 NCHADS can play an important role by providing technical guidance, in coordination with nongovernmental organizations and community members, and by ensuring that a mechanism is in place to provide regular training and technical supervision during data collection. Allowing for technical input from local academic institutions may prove useful.

3.7 In order to improve the set of size estimates available for all risk groups, it is recommended that additional methods such as the "unique object" and "unique event" methods in conjunction with surveys be explored.[39]

Monitoring the quality of HIV programmes

NCHADS has rolled out two quality-improvement methodologies that aim to create a culture of evidence-based quality improvement among continuum of care (CoC) teams. Beginning in 2008, NCHADS, with support from partners, has trained 35 of 62 sites providing care for those with opportunistic infections (OIs)/ART in the use of the continuous quality improvement (CQI) system. As part of CQI, CoC teams track indicators related to mortality, quality of services and prevention, and provide follow-up to address any problem identified. NCHADS has also adopted the WHO HIV drug resistance early warning indicators (EWIs), a set of service quality indicators related to the potential development of HIV drug resistance, which overlap to some extent with the CQI indicators. NCHADS has also developed cohort analysis to estimate levels of retention and survival for patients in treatment. All three efforts – CQI, EWI and cohort analysis – draw primarily on the same OI/ART record and/or database and aim to improve care and treatment outcomes through evidence-based decision-making. CoC teams of provincial health departments rely on NCHADS and CDC (at seven CQI sites) to carry out the analysis. Leadership for these initiatives within NCHADS is divided across research, surveillance and data management units.

In some provinces, such as Battambang, provincial health department directors have developed their own analysis to enable more frequent updating of the CQI indicators. However, this is not systematic, and sustaining and improving capacity for CQI requires additional investments. There is a desire at the national and local levels to decentralize analysis, allowing local teams greater flexibility in applying the CQI and EWI systems. A challenge for NCHADS has been conducting follow-up and supervision for local CoC teams as often as planned due to budgetary limitations.

Community interventions, including outreach, prevention, support for orphans and vulnerable children, and linkage of key-affected populations and people living with HIV to testing and care, are monitored through output indicators such as numbers of meetings, contacts, referrals and services delivered. Efforts are under way to standardize these indicators. Key challenges include double-counting of the same individual across service providers and accurate coverage estimates, given the variability in mapping size estimates.

The current quality-improvement systems and monitoring of community efforts are useful; however, the reasons for loss to follow-up at different stages of the cascade are not systematically investigated and are not well understood.

Recommendations

3.8 Potential gains in efficiency could be explored by consolidating the CQI and EWI indicators in a single set of quality-monitoring indicators and by unifying analysis, training and follow-up functions under one NCHADS unit to avoid duplication. It is suggested that CQI's unique emphasis on CoC team meetings and follow-up be retained under the new, consolidated system. While technically distinct, if the findings from cohort analysis are made available more regularly to CoC teams, they can be reviewed together with the quality indicators, thus providing a more complete picture of trends in patient outcomes.

3.9 It is suggested that a plan with concrete steps to decentralize analysis to the provincial health department and operational district be developed, with increased training and coordination by NCHADS and phased roll-out, beginning with high-burden areas.

3.10 A mechanism to regularly review existing evidence of loss to follow-up along the services cascade is recommended in order to develop targeted qualitative assessments to identify reasons for loss to follow up. Assessments may focus on links in the cascade where existing evidence indicates potential problems.

Monitoring linkages along the services cascade: the need for a unique identifier

Considerable progress has been made by NCHADS in deploying health management information systems (HMISs) to routinely capture information on individual health services. Data systems for voluntary counselling and testing, and services for OI/ART, TB, STI and PMTCT are in place; however, they operate independently of one another. Regular monitoring of linkages along the CoC, for example, from voluntary counselling and testing to services for OI/ART, is not conducted due to the absence of a unique identifier to link patient records across the separate data systems. Similarly, it is not currently possible to monitor linkages in key-affected populations from outreach to testing, care and treatment services because identifiers from outreach are not compatible with those used in the health services.

This also limits the ability to use programme data to identify the risks associated with new infections. To address these limitations, NCHADS is examining three unique identifiers for use in the health services and community outreach:

- In May 2013, NCHADS began piloting fingerprint readers at OI/ART and related health services in Battambang province with support from CDC.
- A national health identification card, including a unique identifier (ID) code, is being rolled out by the MOH with support from the University Research Company. The card is expected to be functioning in 57 operational districts by September 2013 and could allow for de-duplicating of records and linkage within the HIV health services. The health identification card is part of the national health information system, which is in place at hospitals nationwide and some health centres.
- Finally, Flagship Project is piloting an identification code using the individual's sex, birth place and birth year, as well as parents' initials for use in community outreach. This code could conceivably be used at health facilities as well, thus providing a single unique identifier consistent across community and health services.

An effective and sustainable solution to the unique identifier problem will need to accommodate individuals who access a number of services simultaneously (for instance, a person with HIV who also has TB and practices sex work should have a single identifier used by NCHADS, CENAT and community outreach organizations).

Confidentiality and privacy protection should be given careful consideration in the current efforts to personalize sensitive information with a view to strengthening monitoring of the continuum of prevention, care and treatment, and improving partner referral, contact tracing and community mapping. These efforts should be in accordance with and supported by the 2002 national HIV law. Ethically and technically sound operational research should be undertaken to establish the benefits of these measures to individual and public health as well as the risks of infringements on confidentiality and privacy. Such evaluations should *precede* implementation and actively involve the participation of people living with HIV and affected communities. The creation of new databases that store personal health information should also be accompanied by complaint and redressal mechanisms applicable to breaches of confidentiality – whether inadvertent or deliberate – that can be particularly harmful for women, children and key-affected populations.

Recommendations

3.11 NCHADS' efforts to develop a combination of unique identifier systems across the continuum of prevention, care and treatment services are well founded. Establishing well-defined criteria to guide discussion among stakeholders and the eventual selection of a method for introducing a combination of unique identifier systems is recommended (*see* Box 4).

3.12 The review team wishes to draw the attention of the MOH, NCHADS, service providers and civil society to the need for ensuring the protection of privacy and confidentiality, along with the creation of complaint and redressal mechanisms. These mechanisms should be prepared to respond to possible breaches of confidentiality of personal data, as new data management systems are being designed for the purpose of tracking people living with HIV throughout the continuum of prevention, care and treatment.

> **Box 4: Recommended criteria for selection among various unique identifier systems**
>
> An effective and sustainable solution to the unique identifier problem aims to ensure:
>
> (1) a relatively short time for roll-out to reach national coverage, given the pressing need to assess and improve linkages;
> (2) operational feasibility across the range of field conditions;
> (3) minimal recurring equipment and maintenance costs, given the need to achieve more with less over the short term and long term;
> (4) confidentiality protection and acceptability to people living with HIV and to the affected community, especially to the most hidden and stigmatized groups;
> (5) compatibility between two systems (i.e. unique identifier for community outreach and for health facility-based system);
> (6) to the extent possible, the ability to apply the identifier retroactively, in order to provide a historical baseline assessment of linkage across services;
> (7) an identifier that is unique "enough" for public health purposes, while accepting some degree of error as inevitable.

Putting it all together: drawing up the epidemic profile

NCHADS and partners' strong surveillance studies in key-affected populations and programmatic data systems in place at STI clinics, HIV testing sites, and care and treatment facilities provide the raw data necessary to improve understanding of the epidemic both at the national and local levels. A simple example of this is the use of data from routine STI reporting to identify a recent upward trend in genital ulcers in men who have sex with men in Phnom Penh (*see* Section 4). Such an analysis combined with trends in prevention outreach, testing utilization by risk groups, characteristics of individuals with recent HIV diagnoses, effectiveness of treatment among people with HIV, and trends in prevalence and incidence from surveillance studies and routine testing – to name a few – could do much to characterize the sources of new HIV and STI infections both nationally and locally. Yet, these data are not routinely brought together to describe epidemic patterns and identify strengths and weaknesses in programmes. Developing national and local epidemic and response profiles, beginning with those geographical areas most affected by the epidemic, could provide the strategic information needed to enhance efforts to eliminate new HIV infections.

Recommendation

3.13 It is recommended that profiles of the epidemic and response be developed and regularly updated (annually) through greater and integrated analysis of data from surveillance studies, routine surveillance, community outreach and health services. Characterizing recent changes in the epidemic situation, particularly with respect to new HIV and STI infections, and effectiveness of the response will provide stakeholders with the information they need to improve the targeting of interventions. Both national and local-level profiles need to be considered. A phased roll-out, beginning with profiles for the highest-burden regions or cities/provinces, is recommended.

The recommendations for the area of strategic information are summarized in Box 5. Figure 7 illustrates the data recommended for inclusion in local and national profiles of the epidemic situation in key-affected populations. The epidemic risk profile and data from monitoring of the prevention, care and treatment services cascades feed into an integrated profile of risk and response.

Box 5: A summary of critical action points to strengthen strategic information

Given Cambodia 3.0's ambitious targets to scale up programmes and eliminate new infections, strategic information to guide programmes is becoming increasingly important. It is suggested that NCHADS and its partners strive:
(1) to develop national and local profiles of the epidemic and response through greater analysis of surveillance and programme data, strengthen local estimates from surveillance studies in risk groups, reintroduce incidence testing in surveillance studies and triangulate with prevalence trends in young antenatal women;
(2) to continue efforts to standardize and improve mapping and size estimates for risk groups, and work with NGOs well ahead of future surveillance studies to build in multiple size estimates;
(3) to increase investments in the different approaches to monitoring and improving the quality of care and treatment services (CQI, EWIs for HIV drug resistance and patient cohort analysis), decentralizing analysis and streamlining where possible to reduce cost and triangulate findings;
(4) to regularly review available evidence to identify reasons for loss to follow up along the services cascade;
(5) to ensure an effective and sustainable approach to introducing a unique identifier to monitor the prevention and services cascades, by evaluating the available options according to objective criteria (*see* Box 4).

Figure 7: Profiles of risk and response

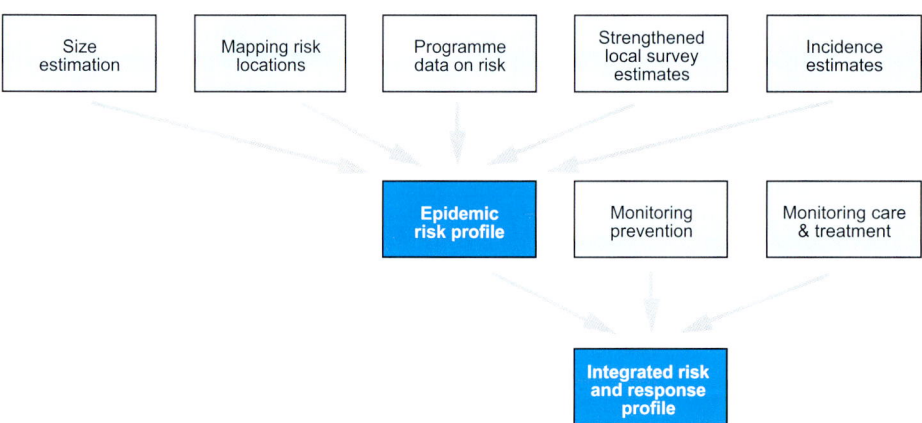

4. Maintaining control of the epidemic

Earlier in its epidemic, Cambodia rolled out effective prevention strategies to control a rapidly spreading epidemic, and then continually adapted them to changing conditions. An important example is the evolving response to sex work where initial implementation of 100% condom use policies in brothel settings was adapted to enable interventions to reach "entertainment workers"– the new term itself reflecting large changes in the organization of sex services – in indirect sex venues, such as bars, massage parlours and karaoke bars. Yet, as the trend towards indirect sex work has continued (Figure 8), new challenges have arisen. These include: (i) increasing intervention coverage and uptake in indirect settings, with many entertainment workers at low or intermediate risk; while (ii) identifying (and prioritizing) smaller numbers of entertainment workers who have many clients and are at substantially higher risk. As discussed in Section 2, this second challenge has become more difficult to address since legislation closed down brothels and previous employees have gone underground to avoid detection.[23]

Figure 8: Changing conditions in sex work in Cambodia, 1995–2010

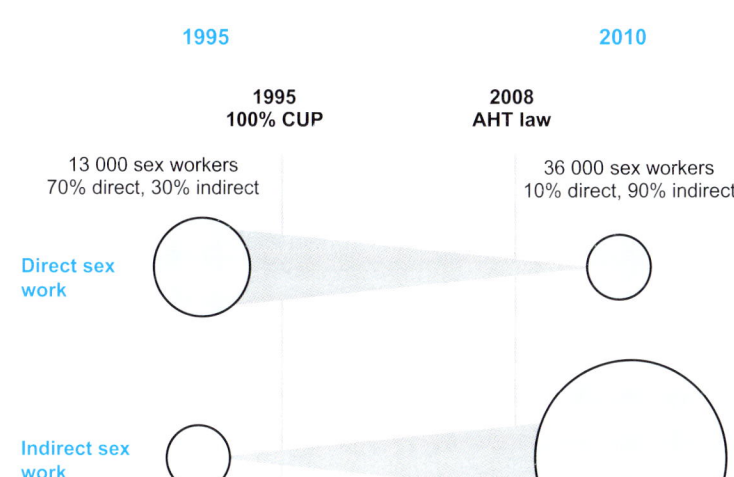

CUP Condom use programme; AHT anti-human trafficking

These challenges apply to other marginalized and vulnerable populations at risk as well, and assume even higher priority in light of the targets to eliminate new HIV infections under Cambodia 3.0.[41] Current efforts are focused on increasing HIV testing, along with standard prevention interventions among defined populations believed to be at greatest risk – entertainment workers, men who have sex with men, transgender persons and drug users (Table 2). However, risk within these populations is highly variable. As a result, many people at relatively low risk are reached and tested frequently, while others at highest risk may fall through the cracks.

The Boosted Continuum of Prevention to Care and Treatment strategy[42] goes beyond this aggregate overview of key populations currently targeted by intervention programmes to document important and overlapping risk behaviours, particularly among specific subgroups. Where reliable data exist, reported risks correlate with higher HIV and/or STI rates.[11,33] Furthermore, recent costing studies strongly support targeting interventions to subpopulations of entertainment workers, drug users, men who have sex with men and transgender persons at highest risk.

The recommendations for strengthening the current response can thus be grouped under several related objectives to ensure that people most at risk for acquiring and transmitting HIV/STI are identified and reached by essential interventions and services. This would also optimize the outcomes and impact of the services provided by improving retention, effectiveness and efficiency at each step of the cascade of services (*See* Box 6).

The first of these is addressed below while the second is discussed later in this section under specific populations and risk settings. HIV testing and optimizing the cascade of services are primarily covered in Section 5 and strategic information in Section 3. In all of these areas, there are important special considerations that apply to marginalized and vulnerable high-risk populations. Some of these, related to enabling environment and confidentiality, have already been addressed in Section 2.

Table 2: Select data on broadly defined populations at risk

Group	Estimated population size	HIV data	STI data	Behavioural and other factors
People who use and inject drugs	Population size of drug users is estimated to be 13 000, including 1300 people who inject drugs (some NGOs consider the actual number to be far higher)	Drug users: 4% overall, 21% among women People who inject drugs: 24% overall, 50% among women	No data	Injecting drug use is thought to be mostly confined to Phnom Penh Condom use with all partners is lower among people who inject drugs than among other users
Men who have sex with men (MSM) and transgender/transsexual persons	2010 estimate 21 327 MSM population (KHANA, FHI) No transgender/transsexual population size estimate	BROS Khmer study (2010) found HIV prevalence of 2.1% among MSM 34% had an HIV test in past year and knew result	Large increase in genital ulcers reported from clinics in Phnom Penh and Battambang during the past year	55.3% and 67.5% consistent condom use by MSM only with male paid partners and male non-paid partners, respectively; 40% of MSM had sex with a female partner in the past year, with female entertainment workers identified as most common sexual partner
Entertainment workers (non-specified)	Estimated near 40 000 (although many in some categories deny selling sex)	13.9% had more than seven clients per week, 4% had fewer than seven clients per week	Largely stable over past decade but recent increase in genital ulcer disease trends	Most entertainment workers live in Phnom Penh (59%), Siem Reap (9%), Battambang (6%) and Banteay Meanchey (4%)
Populations in prisons and other closed settings	Prisons: 15 404[a] inmates (2012), estimated 8% of these are women in detention centres	No data	No data	Anecdotal evidence of sex and drug use in prisons, denied by prison services

[a] This figure differs from that given in the section on closed settings, as different data sources were used.
NGOs nongovernmental organizations

> Box 6: Actions towards reaching those at highest risk for HIV
>
> (1) Sharper epidemiological targeting: reaching those at highest risk.
> (2) Stronger primary prevention: ensuring maximum intervention impact for greatest risk.
> (3) Improved HIV case detection: building trust, promoting and facilitating HIV testing.
> (4) More sustained follow-through: maintain PLHIV within cascade of services.
> (5) More reliable information: to guide the response.

Sharper epidemiological targeting

There is a strong consensus that at this stage of its HIV epidemic, with an eye on elimination of new infections, Cambodia needs to sharpen its epidemiological targeting.[k] The objective should be to reach the remaining pockets of individuals at very high risk of acquiring HIV/STI and of transmitting infections to new partners (*See* Box 6).

Clear examples of such populations that were investigated during the review are drug-injecting women who sell sex and drug-injecting men who have sex with men and transgender persons. These populations are concentrated in Phnom Penh – where over 85% of injecting drug users are believed to live – as well as Battambang, Poipet and a few other, mainly urban, areas. Many spend time in detention centres or prison, and are thereby at very high risk for HIV. In Phnom Penh alone, over 100 individuals in each group are currently known to peer educators. Yet, multiple informants from community and service providers estimate that only about half of them have any contact with existing services. Such a gap may easily account for several hundred new HIV infections each year.

On the other side of the spectrum, important resources are much less effectively allocated to reach large populations at relatively low risk of HIV/STI infection. These may include casino or restaurant workers, for example. Other large populations with a range of risk – karaoke and beer promoters, for example – should be segmented where possible and targeted differentially according to likely risk (do they sell sex? If so, how often?). Peer educators are in the best position to assess such risk and should be trained and supported to focus their efforts on those with the highest number of clients/partners and multiple risk factors (for example, injecting drug and selling sex).

---

[k] The increasing difficulty of this work should be acknowledged and planned for. As prevalence decreases and HIV transmission approaches elimination, investments in detection and prevention of new infections will yield diminishing returns. The final phase of disease elimination is the most challenging and difficult to sustain.

Figure 9: Sharper epidemiological targeting to optimize "boosted" continuum of prevention to care and treatment

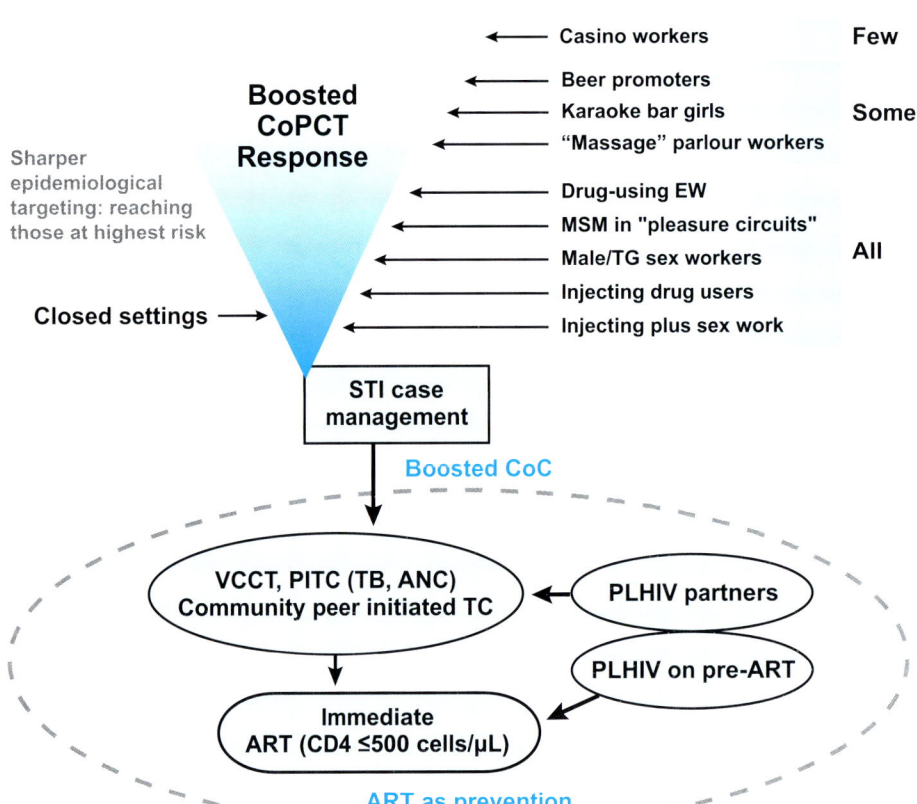

ANC antenatal care; ART antiretroviral treatment; CoC continuum of care; CoPCT continuum of prevention to care and treatment; EW entertainment worker; MSM men who have sex with men; PITC provider-initiated testing and counselling; PLHIV people living with AIDS; STI sexually transmitted infection; TB tuberculosis; TG transgender persons; VCCT voluntary and confidential counselling and testing

An important prerequisite for reaching marginalized populations at highest risk is to remove structural barriers that may drive them underground. The major barrier cited by all partners involved in outreach and services to vulnerable groups is the heightened fear of the police (*see* Section 2) during recent years, following the commune safety policy (and the earlier anti-trafficking law).

Recommendations

4.1 Outreach and services to drug-injecting women and drug-injecting men who have sex with men and transgender persons in Phnom Penh and other identified urban areas should be prioritized within the Boosted Continuum of Prevention to Care and Treatment strategy as a first step to ensuring high coverage of these key populations. Ensuring a more enabling environment and peer/community engagement is critical to the success of these efforts.

4.2 NCHADS should consider establishing an epidemiological rapid response mechanism following the principles of standard communicable disease outbreak investigation and control, with resources to investigate pockets of potential high incidence (HIV, STI and related infections), and to quickly strengthen the response in such areas (*see* Box 7).

Box 7: Rapid response mechanisms

Rapid response mechanisms use standard epidemiological methods for outbreak investigation to identify pockets of proven or potential HIV transmission, and to immediately strengthen the prevention response in those areas. The work can be carried out by a small NCHADS team with basic training in field epidemiology (for example, Field Epidemiology Training Programme) operating with sufficient resources to investigate and strengthen interventions where needed. The purpose of such a team is to look widely for evidence of transmission or weak programme implementation, investigate the potential for transmission in such areas, and mobilize human and financial resources to strengthen the response. Rapid response teams thus have three main functions:
- enhanced vigilance of potential transmission, risk behaviours and underperforming programmes;
- targeted investigation of outbreaks, new pockets of risk and assessment of the adequacy of the response; and
- immediate strengthening of interventions (local microplanning).

Entertainment workers

Cambodia is internationally recognized for having halted and reversed its HIV epidemic by interrupting transmission in sex work. Conditions have changed markedly, however, during the past decade and new strategies are needed to prevent infections in much smaller and more hidden high-risk sex work networks than were reached earlier.

All government and nongovernmental organization partners working with entertainment workers agree that it is difficult to identify the key-affected individuals among the many entertainment workers currently targeted. As a result, interventions are spread widely (not efficiently) across populations with varying risk patterns. Exceptions were noted in some venues where sex took place on site or entertainment workers acknowledged large numbers of partners. Interventions in such settings were stronger when real peer educators were chosen from among the target population, thus maintaining a permanent presence to promote prevention and recommended clinic visits. Involvement of peers in outreach has also enabled community-based nongovernmental organizations to identify entertainment workers with overlapping drug-use and sex-work risks, particularly in heavily affected areas of Phnom Penh (note that nongovernmental organizations working with drug users appear to be better able to identify those with overlapping risk than those working with entertainment workers or men who have sex with men/transgender persons). Shifting some resources from large low-risk populations to more intensive peer-based outreach and interventions will increase effectiveness, as is planned under the Boosted Continuum of Prevention to Care and Treatment strategy. If existing structural barriers can also be improved (as recommended in Section 2), such efforts could avert several hundred new HIV infections per year.

Recommendations

4.3 The Boosted Continuum of Prevention to Care and Treatment strategy should strengthen outreach activities that intensify interventions for subpopulations of entertainment workers at greatest vulnerability and risk. These populations include (i) entertainment workers with a large number of sexual partners (more than seven partners a week), (ii) entertainment workers at venues where sex takes place on site (quasi-brothels, guesthouses, massage parlours, etc.), (iii) drug-using entertainment workers and (iv) non-establishment-based entertainment workers in settings of potential high vulnerability (streets, truck stops, etc.).

4.4 In addition to the above, it is recommendeded that hidden high-transmission sex-work networks be investigated through formative and intervention-linked research, utilizing peer networks and proven epidemiological methods (snowball sampling, rapid response methods, etc.).

Men who have sex with men and transgender persons

The challenge of identifying and reaching those who are at greatest risk also applies to men who have sex with men and transgender persons. While HIV prevalence among men who have sex with men remains relatively low at 2.3% in Cambodia, the risk of HIV acquisition and transmission is high among some subgroups, as well as among transgender persons.[33] Risk is also high and varies by subgroup, as documented in the Boosted Continuum of Prevention to Care and Treatment strategy, and overlaps considerably with wider sex-work and drug-using networks. Peer outreach workers and nongovernmental organizations working with men who have sex with men and transgender persons report high rates of sex partner change among two main groups – those who sell sex and men in non-paying "pleasure circuits", such as those who frequent saunas and bars in Phnom Penh. Condom use is reportedly variable, particularly among men who have sex with men and transgender persons who use drugs. In the past year, STI symptoms, most commonly genital sores, were reported by about half of the men who have sex with men surveyed.[33] NCHADS recently noted a fourfold increase in genital ulcers reported mainly from four clinics in Phnom Penh, which appears to be spreading among other men (who do not have sex with men) and entertainment workers.[i] Taken together, these data indicate that many unprotected high-risk exposures are taking place, and suggest that HIV may be spreading through the same overlapping sexual and drug-injecting networks, where existing prevention efforts are inadequate.

Recommendations

4.5 Existing interventions among men who have sex with men should be strengthened under the Boosted Continuum of Prevention to Care and Treatment strategy. Focusing on men who sell sex and men in non-paying "pleasure circuits" (frequenting saunas, for example) with large numbers of partners, as well as drug-using men who have sex with men is suggested. Strengthening the link to STI services (for routine check-ups and syphilis screening) would help to control the rising incidence of ulcerative STIs in this population. (Monitoring the rising incidence of STIs acts as an indicator of the effectiveness of prevention efforts.)

4.6 Outreach and peer interventions to transgender persons, especially those who use drugs, along with appropriate services and follow up, are an immediate priority, while more complete mapping, size estimates and biobehavioural data on higher-risk subpopulations are carried out to guide the response.

---

[i] NCHADS routine STI surveillance data. Presentation available at: http://www.nchads.org/Publication/dissemination/STI%20Sentinel%20Survey%202011_eng.pdf

People who use drugs

Integrated behavioural and biological surveillance data estimates from 2007 indicate that the number of persons who injected drugs in Cambodia was estimated at 1100–1700 individuals, of whom 15% were women. Heroin was the main drug injected, followed by ice (crystal methamphetamine). It was estimated that 85% of all injectors and 86% of all heroin injectors were located in Phnom Penh.[44] The mean age of the injectors was 25 years and HIV prevalence was 24.4%. The current (2012) HIV prevalence among injectors, as estimated by the methadone maintenance treatment programme, is 21%, while the prevalence of TB is just under 7%. The risk of TB/HIV coinfection is of concern. The prevalence of hepatitis B virus infection among HIV-infected people who inject drugs is 35%, while the prevalence of hepatitis virus / HIV coinfection is 82%. To date, Cambodia has no response to viral hepatitis beyond diagnosis.

The availability of effective interventions for people who inject drugs in Cambodia is limited to Phnom Penh. This is consistent with the current epidemiology of injecting in the country. Compared with the estimated population of people who inject drugs, however, coverage is inadequate. Two nongovernmental organizations are licensed to provide needle and syringe programmes in conjunction with two other nongovernmental organizations, dividing Phnom Penh geographically to minimize overlap. These same nongovernmental organizations provide referrals for methadone maintenance treatment and this constitutes a strength. In 2011, the number of syringes supplied per person who injects drugs was 120 (0.3/day).[m,45] However, the reported injecting frequency is three to four times daily. Methadone maintenance treatment has been available at one site (Department of Mental Health, Khmer Soviet Hospital) since 2010 (see Box 8). While the programme has cumulatively treated 290 individuals, only 150 were in the programme in 2012, underscoring the fact that low retention was an issue, in combination with a consistently low intake rate of new patients. The mean dosage of methadone was 79 mg, which is within the recommended therapeutic range. The review team noted that participants in the methadone programme reported substantial reductions in heroin injecting frequency. The high drop-out rate is probably due to access issues attributed (by both staff and clients) to a solitary dispensing site with limited hours, an adverse policing environment and no provision for "take-home" doses.[n]

Recommendations

4.7 It is recommended that the MOH, through the National Program of Mental Health, NCHADS and other relevant partners, scale up the coverage of needle–syringe programmes and related services to people who inject drugs across Phnom Penh, utilizing secondary needle–syringe programme distribution (through networks of people who inject drugs) and working with local authorities to improve access and reach hidden populations.

4.8 Scale up methadone maintenance treatment programmes within Phnom Penh to ensure wider coverage. It would be advisable to focus initially on rapidly expanding the existing service while maximizing retention in treatment through provision of take-home dosing, and lowering the threshold for drop-outs who restart treatment.

---

[m] Nineteen hundred people who inject drugs (NCHADS 2007 estimate) received over 228 362 needles and syringes.

[n] Take-home dosing permits dispensing multiple doses to participants when circumstances (work, travel home for holidays, etc.) would otherwise result in treatment interruptions.

> **Box 8: Methadone maintenance treatment**
>
> Methadone maintenance treatment has been offered at one site in Phnom Penh since 2010. Of 290 registered clients, 271 (93%) have accepted HIV testing and counselling. Of these, 57 (21%) are HIV-positive. Among these HIV-positive persons, 32 are active clients on methadone maintenance treatment, and 28 are on ART. Reported benefits of the programme include decreases in drug-related arrests and episodes of overdose, and a marked reduction in injecting frequency among adherent clients.
>
> However, access to the methadone maintenance treatment programme is limited and the programme drop-out rate has increased from the early low levels. Of the 290 enrolled, only 150 are currently active clients. This is attributed partly to legal barriers (village/commune safety), and partly to mobility, access and job-related conflicts (having to dose during working hours). Previous proposals to address these issues and improve access, such as provision of take-home doses, earlier and more flexible opening hours, and a satellite site, have not yet been implemented. Peer-based outreach should also be strengthened. In addition, a new initiative with the General Department of Prisons to train prison medical staff may create opportunities to introduce opioid substitution therapy in prisons through mobile services or on-site methadone maintenance treatment.
>
> Potential demand is believed to be high – it is estimated that participation in the methadone maintenance treatment programme could be doubled to more than 300. With higher numbers, the programme would be more cost effective – the estimated average daily cost per user would decrease from US$ 4 to US$ 2 per day with 300 active participants, equivalent to programme costs elsewhere in the Region.

Closed settings

As of the end of June 2011, there were 15 325 prisoners° and detainees in 28 prisons across the country, of which 1209 (7.9%) were women. Overcrowding is common across the sector, while adequate nutrition remains an issue. During the first six months of 2011, the General Department of Prisons, Ministry of Interior, reported 301 HIV cases and 1323 suspected TB cases, of whom 133 were confirmed to have TB, and 24 cases (18%) TB/HIV coinfection. It is unclear whether all inmates were screened for TB and HIV, though many have been. The review team visited Svay Rieng provincial prison, where at least 12 TB cases had been identified out of the 301 inmates, though results were not available for all 52 persons suspected of having TB. HIV screening was not made available to inmates. Infection control measures are not possible in that overcrowded prison. TB and HIV data were not available for the drug rehabilitation centres visited by the review team.

Prison personnel deny that sexual intercourse occurs within the prison sector (especially male to male).[30] In 2012, NCHADS developed standard operating procedures for the prevention, care and treatment of HIV, STI and TB/HIV in collaboration with CENAT. The review team noted that HIV screening on entry and intermittent mobile TB screening were available in a number of prisons, and have recently been introduced in at least one drug rehabilitation centre. However, screening appears not to be consistent with standard operating procedures. In particular, the offer of HIV and TB screening to inmates and staff is irregular. There is no follow-up for residents of drug rehabilitation centres when they move back to the community, so rehabilitation and recidivism rates are unclear.

° This figure differs from that in Table 2 on closed settings as different data sources were used.

Recommendations

4.9 The Ministry of Interior, through the General Department of Prisons, should introduce HIV prevention interventions, including the provision of condoms, as a priority in closed settings. For prison inmates who inject drugs, it is suggested that harm reduction including opioid substitution therapy be made available, with referral to services in the community on release from prison, ensuring continuity of care for those on opioid substitution treatment.

4.10 Considering the commendable introduction of active TB case-finding in closed settings, the review team recommends the offer of provider-initiated voluntary HIV testing and counselling by all prison health posts to prison inmates, as described in the 2012 *Standard operating procedures for HIV, STI and TB/HIV prevention, care, treatment and support in prisons (and correctional centres) in Cambodia*.[46] It is advised that ART, isoniazid preventive therapy, TB and STI treatment (in accordance with national standard operating procedures) be provided to all coinfected patients. Infection control measures would also need to be introduced and prison personnel trained accordingly.

STI services

Following early increases of condom use in sex work, large reductions in STIs (syphilis, chancroid, gonorrhoea and chlamydia) were measured among sex workers, high-risk men and pregnant women. Prevalence rates of common curable STIs declined markedly in Cambodia between 1996 and 2001 but have plateaued over the past decade. Subsequent STI surveys in 2005 and 2010 have not shown further reduction, and STI case reports routinely collected from government and nongovernmental STI clinics since 2006 also show a levelling off of STI incidence at intermediate levels. In fact, the incidence of ulcerative STIs actually appears to be increasing among both men and entertainment workers. More recently, NCHADS identified a large increase in genital ulcer disease cases among men who have sex with men, which was reported by a few STI clinics in Phnom Penh (Figure 10). These data indicate that sexual transmission of STIs is taking place, at least in some areas, and that prevention efforts need to be strengthened. The increase in sexual transmission in these sexual networks suggests a high risk of ongoing HIV transmission. Routine STI case reports thus need to be closely monitored to assess the prevention response and pinpoint areas where interventions need to be strengthened. As recommended during the earlier implementation of the 100% condom use programme, routinely interviewing all new STI male patients about the locations of recent sexual contacts would provide information that could be used to identify venues where condom use needs boosting. In addition, syphilis testing needs to be routinely offered to entertainment workers, men who have sex with men and transgender persons every six months, and prevalence and incidence trends monitored.

Recommendations

4.11 The national network of STI clinics, which performs a critical prevention function for key-affected populations, should be reinforced. In order to ensure user-friendliness and unimpeded access to services, upgradation of services would be needed. NCHADS could upgrade and consider expanding the STI services (Family Health Clinics), strengthening capacity and increasing user-friendliness and access for key-affected populations. Building the capacity of Family Health Clinics would help them to function as the local "eyes" of the "rapid response mechanism" (*see* recommendation 4.2 and Box 7), and take an active role in monitoring "hotspots" and community-based interventions, investigating outbreaks and strengthening the response.

4.12 Strengthening the analysis and use of routine STI data is needed to pinpoint areas where increasing STI rates indicate that the prevention response may be weak, and this information could be used to inform the work of the rapid response mechanism described above. Information obtained from new male STI patients about venues of recent sexual exposure could be used to strengthen prevention work in those areas.

4.13 It is recommended that the role and performance of STI control in the overall response to HIV be reviewed. Strengthening the capacity for STI control is advised in targeted prevention efforts (through routine check-ups of entertainment workers, men who have sex with men and transgender persons), routine monitoring and surveillance of sexual transmission trends. Priority indicators for prevention of sexual transmission would need to include trend analysis of male STI case reports (genital ulcers and urethral discharge), as well as monitoring of syphilis prevalence and incidence among entertainment workers, men who have sex with men and transgender persons.

Figure 10: Genital ulcers among men who have sex with men and other male STI patients, NCHADS routine STI clinic case reports, 2010–2012

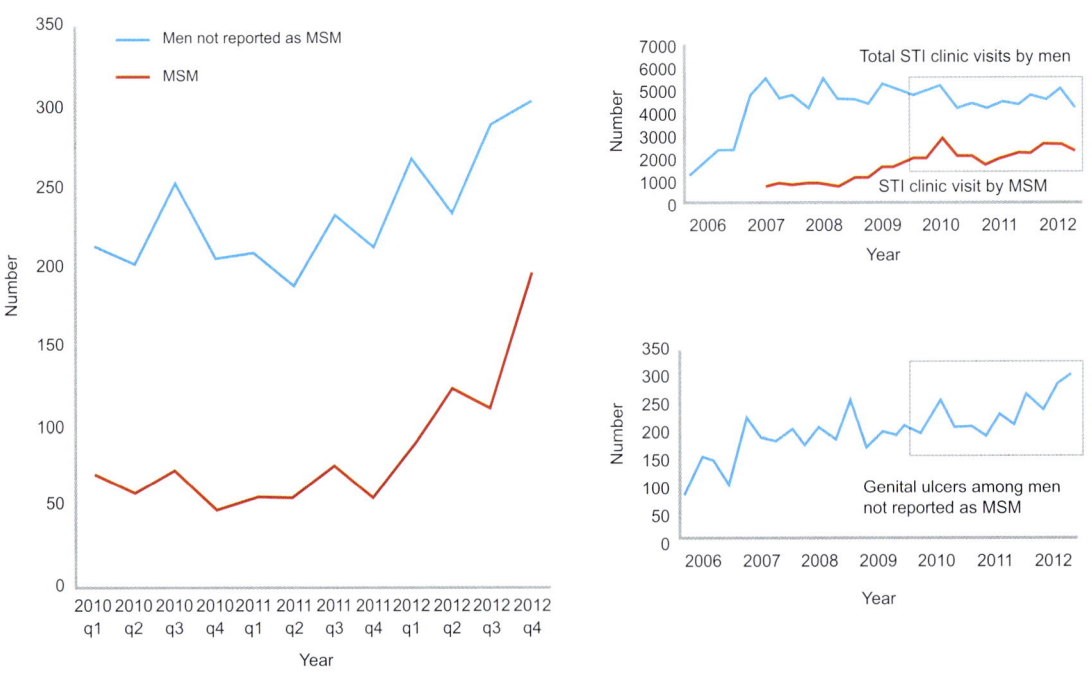

MSM men who have sex with men; STI sexually transmitted infection
Remark: The blue line in the figure at left is a zoom-in of the blue line from 2010 to 2012 in the figure bottom-right.

5. Optimizing the cascade of interventions: HIV testing, linkages to prevention, care and treatment

When ARVs are effective in reducing viral load, they can greatly reduce morbidity and mortality, and a person's likelihood of transmitting HIV through sexual transmission and from mother to child.[35] Harnessing the dual benefit of ARVs for both treatment and prevention depends on the uptake of HIV testing, linkage and retention of HIV-positive individuals in HIV care and treatment, and suppression of viral load.[47] The aim is to increase the number of people living with HIV on treatment and reduce the number of individuals lost at each step of the HIV treatment cascade (Figure 11). The country is poised to implement the elimination of mother-to-child transmission initiative based on the new "B+" strategy, which offers immediate ART for all HIV-positive pregnant and breastfeeding women, regardless of clinical and immunological staging,[48] linking prevention services for key-affected populations[49] and earlier treatment for prevention for HIV-positive partners in serodiscordant couples.[50] One of the key elements of the new conceptual framework is the evolution of HIV testing strategies, where one rapid HIV screening test is done in the community and at primary care-level health facilities and, if screened positive, confirmatory testing is done at a voluntary counselling and testing facility co-located with pre-ART/ART services. This is expected to substantially streamline the referral procedure and reduce drop-out from HIV diagnosis to enrolment in the pre-ART/ART services.

Figure 11: HIV treatment service cascade[51]

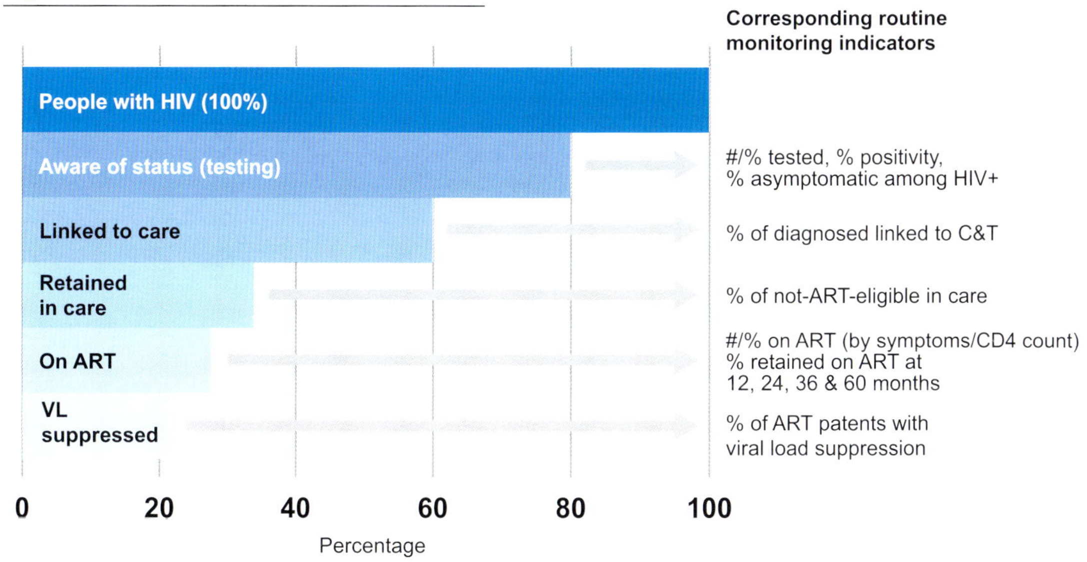

Cascade stage	Corresponding routine monitoring indicators
People with HIV (100%)	
Aware of status (testing)	#/% tested, % positivity, % asymptomatic among HIV+
Linked to care	% of diagnosed linked to C&T
Retained in care	% of not-ART-eligible in care
On ART	#/% on ART (by symptoms/CD4 count) % retained on ART at 12, 24, 36 & 60 months
VL suppressed	% of ART patents with viral load suppression

ART antiretroviral treatment; C&T care and treatment; VL viral load

This requires robust services and monitoring systems that allow for appropriate case-finding, registration of baseline data, longitudinal follow up of individuals, and the regular analysis and evaluation of data to identify leakages in the cascade, allowing for course corrections.

Expanding HIV testing and counselling

Remarkable progress has been made in expanding voluntary confidential counselling and HIV testing. Testing occurs in a wide range of settings, including antenatal care (55.1%), self-referrals or walk-ins at voluntary counselling and testing centres (29.9%), as well as a smaller number of referrals from nongovernmental organizations/home-based care programmes (5.2%), TB (2.4%), STI (1.2%) and other services.

The first testing site was established in 1995.[16] Access to voluntary counselling and testing sites expanded rapidly from 12 in 2000. By 2005, most operational districts had sites for voluntary counselling and testing. By the end of October 2012, there were 253 sites with the majority (229) in the public sector and a few (24) in the nongovernment sector. Voluntary counselling and testing is now available at approximately one in five health centres. In addition, provider-initiated HIV testing for TB patients and pregnant women is available in most health centres through health staff providing TB and maternal and child health services. Recently, voluntary counselling and testing has included community-based testing for key populations at intervention sites.

In 2011, NCHADS reported that there were 704 979 clients who opted for voluntary counselling and testing, of whom 99.9% accepted HIV testing. The proportion of women compared to men among voluntary counselling and testing clients increased from 64% in 2009 to 69% in 2012 (Figure 12). At present, the percentage of newly diagnosed cases of HIV infection is low, at approximately 1.8% of self-referred and TB patients, and less than 1% of pregnant women.[53] However, it is not entirely clear how the current system can report the number of individuals tested in the absence of unique health identifiers (*see* Box 9).

Box 9: Monitoring the number of individuals tested and re-tested

Reporting on the number of new HIV diagnoses and the percentage of positive HIV tests among those presenting for testing during the period should take into account each individual only once, regardless of the number of re-tests for that individual during the period. Individuals testing negative on all tests should be entered as a single negative entry; individuals testing positive on at least one test should be entered as a single positive entry. Similarly, it is important that the monitoring system determines how many of those individuals who screen positive follow up with confirmatory testing at the ART site and are confirmed, as well as how many of those individuals who are confirmed cases actually enrol in care and treatment. This not only requires a unique identifier but re-testing should also be reflected in the recording and reporting forms.

Figure 12: Number of people who had an HIV test, by gender, Cambodia, 2009–2011[54]

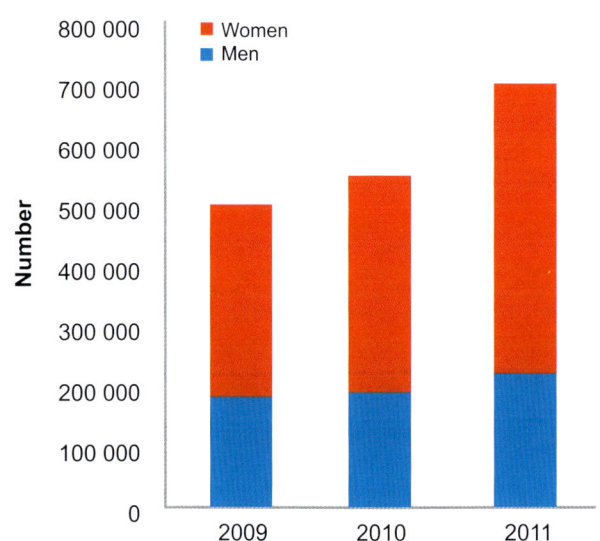

Since 2009, Cambodia's national HIV programme has promoted provider-initiated testing and counselling.[54] It is promoted in antenatal care, STI and TB clinical care settings. By 2011, provider-initiated testing and counselling for pregnant women and TB cases had been expanded to most health centres in all 77 operational districts. HIV testing and counselling, and indeed all HIV primary care, are provided free, as mandated by law.

Targeted HIV testing focusing on key populations and partners of HIV-positive individuals is already being conducted, and further expansion would be feasible and allow for sharper epidemiological targeting of interventions. The field team that visited Battambang was informed about the pilot to roll out finger-prick testing for HIV in the community. The results were not available at the time of the review. The further decentralization of HIV testing will be helpful in this process, such as expanding finger-prick HIV testing by mobilizing nongovernmental organizations and peer outreach workers who reach and serve key-affected populations.

This may also be a good opportunity for trained outreach workers to continue to support their clients, even after they are found to be HIV positive, to access care and help retain them in care.

Integrated HIV and syphilis testing in pregnant women

Antenatal HIV testing

Free, routine, opt-out antenatal HIV testing is offered in almost all health facilities that provide antenatal care. This includes antenatal care at primary-level health facilities, where HIV testing may be available directly on site, or via blood specimen referral. In all settings, individual pre-test counselling is provided for antenatal care clients, and verbal informed consent is obtained. The newly revised Linked Response plan[p,55,56] entitled "Boosted Linked Response" introduced the use of the triple rapid test methodology (first test: Determine HIV1/2, second rapid test: Stat-Pak and the third rapid test: Uni-Gold), which will be used at voluntary counselling and testing sites. In health centres without voluntary counseling and testing, following pre-test counseling, blood specimens are sent to health facilities with voluntary counseling and testing. HIV test results are delivered with post-test counselling after one week in antenatal care settings. But if voluntary counselling and testing is available on site, clients are referred to it on the same day for confirmation and the result is given there. Pregnant women with a negative test result undergo a risk assessment; if a transmission risk is identified, re-testing is recommended in three months. As part of the Cambodia 3.0 initiative, the first screening test in antenatal care will use a finger-prick rapid HIV test at health centres without a laboratory, and the person is referred to a voluntary counselling and testing site co-located with pre-ART/ART services for confirmation.

Antenatal syphilis testing

Syphilis testing has been linked with routine antenatal HIV screening. The specimen used for HIV testing at a given site, whether it is finger-stick blood or venous blood, is also used for initial syphilis screening, which is conducted using a rapid test. Women who have an initial positive test result are referred to one of the 32 STI or nongovernmental organization clinics for a confirmatory rapid plasma reagin (RPR) test and, if necessary, treatment. At present, there are 32 STI clinics in 22 provinces which are equipped to provide syphilis treatment. Of the 374 986 pregnant women attending their first antenatal care visit, 184 878 pregnant women (49%) had a syphilis test. Of those, 0.07% (134) tested positive for syphilis by the RPR method (Table 3).

---

[p] Linked Response is a strategy implemented at operational district level to increase the coverage of HIV prevention, care and treatment, and reproductive health, including maternal health and PMTCT services by strengthening patients' referrals and follow up within and between community-based organizations and various facility-based services.

Table 3: Antenatal syphilis testing, 2012

% of women accessing antenatal care services who were tested for syphilis at the first antenatal visit	49.3% (184 878/374 986)
% of antenatal care attendees who were tested and positive for syphilis	0.07% (134/184 878)
% of antenatal care attendees positive for syphilis who received treatment	98.5% (132/134)

Source: Cambodia global AIDS reporting, 2013 (Ref: Excel sheets final consolidated 4 April 2013)

Couples and partner testing and counselling

In 2012, 65 491 male partners (17%) of the 374 986 pregnant women attending antenatal care were tested for HIV. From January to September 2012, 99 (0.19%) of the 51 115 men tested in antenatal care sites were found to be HIV infected. This is very similar to the 0.3% rate of HIV infection in pregnant women in 2012. It is not known how many of the male partners of the 1153 HIV-positive pregnant women identified in antenatal care in that year came for testing and, by design, there is no linking of test results between a specific pregnant woman and her partner. Thus, it is not currently possible to readily identify discordant couples for intensive prevention services unless individual providers have this information.

Moreover, in some sites, such as in Svay Rieng and Banteay Meanchey provinces, partner testing includes partners of HIV-negative pregnant women. Given the low HIV prevalence in the country, this does not seem to make best use of limited resources.

Other issues identified during the review included lack of voluntary disclosure of HIV-positive status to sexual partners and families in some sites visited by the team in Battambang and Phnom Penh. In Svay Rieng hospital, the counselling and testing of a pregnant woman and her partner took place at the same time, although in different rooms, and by a woman and a man, respectively.

Targeted HIV re-testing during the window period

It appears that many, if not most, people who test negative are told to return for another test in three to six months. A focused strategy of re-testing those with initial indeterminate results (a positive screening test but not confirmed by further tests), or those with higher risk factors, might be more worthwhile.

Confidentiality of HIV status

Safeguards to ensure confidentiality have been in place since 2002.[22] The culture in Cambodia emphasizes confidentiality; the term in Khmer means "maintaining secrets". An earlier WHO mission in January 2013 commented that "this emphasis may be counterproductive" as couples testing and counselling and voluntary disclosure to the partner improve retention in care and adherence to treatment.[57] The mission report stated that when there is much emphasis in voluntary counselling and testing or ART services on "maintaining secrets", it is easy to understand why clients and patients do not disclose their status to their partners and families. This atmosphere of secrecy also seems to extend within and between services, as what is learnt in voluntary counselling and testing is not communicated to the ART provider and community outreach workers who refer high-risk persons for testing are rarely informed of the test results. Confidentiality of patient information should be maintained for all medical information, including HIV diagnosis and treatment. However, this should not prevent members of the care team from sharing information as needed with other health workers to ensure good care and promote partner testing and expansion of services to partners and family members. As with all medical information, the patient should provide consent regarding with whom medical information may be shared. The concept of "shared confidentiality" has been used in some countries to encourage appropriate sharing of information within the care team and the family.

Earlier diagnosis of HIV status and enrolment to care

Same-day HIV test results are not consistently available across the voluntary counselling and testing sites at different levels of the health services. It may take up to one week to receive a confirmatory HIV test result and about two to four weeks to receive the CD4 count result. In such a situation, persons referred to a voluntary counselling and testing/care centre would have to go there twice: one visit for counselling and testing and, usually, a second visit one week later for obtaining the test result. If positive, the person would be referred to the service providing treatment and care. Psychological, financial and logistic factors may determine if the individual will follow the set process or simply drop out.

Currently, it is difficult to determine whether people testing HIV-positive are tested late, or lost between voluntary counselling and testing and enrolment into ART, since there is no mechanism to actively track this process. There is also no mechanism to ensure that HIV-positive individuals referred from one facility to another actually reach the other service.

It would be useful to understand the reasons for late HIV diagnosis, characteristics of clients and time before presentation to HIV care services – whether these are asymptomatic HIV-infected individuals infected years ago or more recently (median CD4 count at diagnosis could indicate stage of immunological disease progression), or whether they present to the health services and are then denied care or lost to follow up ("missed opportunities"). In addition, it would be important to assess if there are differences in the promptness of HIV diagnosis and/or in the efficiency of referral to treatment among different subpopulations to inform sharper epidemiological targeting. Such differences might be linked to gender, age, risk/vulnerability factors, urban versus rural location or pregnancy status. This knowledge should be derived from focal studies, as readily available data are insufficient to support such analyses.

Recommendations

5.1 Ongoing efforts to decentralize HIV testing (first screening test) and train peer outreach workers, health centre and maternal and child health staff including midwives in conducting voluntary counselling and HIV testing should continue in order to make available same-day test results, link individuals into care and follow them through treatment. Quality management systems will have to be expanded to include community-based testing.

5.2 It is advised that maternal and child health services and NCHADS continue to offer HIV testing to male partners and family members, including children of HIV-positive pregnant women in antenatal settings, and consider expansion of this offer to HIV-positive index persons receiving voluntary counselling and testing and OI/ART care. Putting in place systems to monitor uptake of such testing and linking test results, for example, of partners of HIV-positive index persons, would facilitate intensified HIV prevention for serodiscordant couples.

5.3 The concept of "shared confidentiality" could be considered for application by NCHADS in health-care settings. This would need to be tested and implemented with utmost caution, and monitored and protected. It is advisable for trained health-care workers within and across health facilities from health centre to referral hospital to be aware of the HIV status, co-morbidities and clinical treatment of their patients. This information could be made available to trained treatment supporters with the consent of the client. Likewise, information on follow-up of people living with HIV by the MMM and other self-help groups could be made available to health staff in the same facility to ensure the continuum of care.

5.4 For consenting clients, the role of treatment supporters could be expanded to involve selected trained prevention outreach workers who work with specific key populations (for example, HIV-positive men who have sex with men) to ensure retention in care. As in health-care facilities, this would need to be tested and implemented with utmost caution, and monitored and protected.

5.5 As recommended by WHO, a focused strategy should be developed of re-testing those with indeterminate results (a positive screening test but not confirmed) or those with higher risk rather than re-testing every individual with a negative test result.

Care and treatment for adults, adolescents and children

There has been an impressive scale-up of access to HIV care and ART. By the end of 2012, 48 913 (81%) of the estimated adults and children requiring ART (CD4 count <350 cells/μL) were receiving treatment. Of those on ART, 53% were women and 9% (4595) were children, 46% girls and 54% boys. Current ART services cover 21 out of 24 provinces through 61 clinics (57 public, four private) of which 59 are hospitals and two health centres located in 50 operational districts providing pre-ART and ART care to children, pregnant women and adults. Paediatric pre-ART/ART services are available only in 35 clinics within 33 operational districts.[58]

Figure 13: Distribution of PLHIV in care cascade, Cambodia (2012)

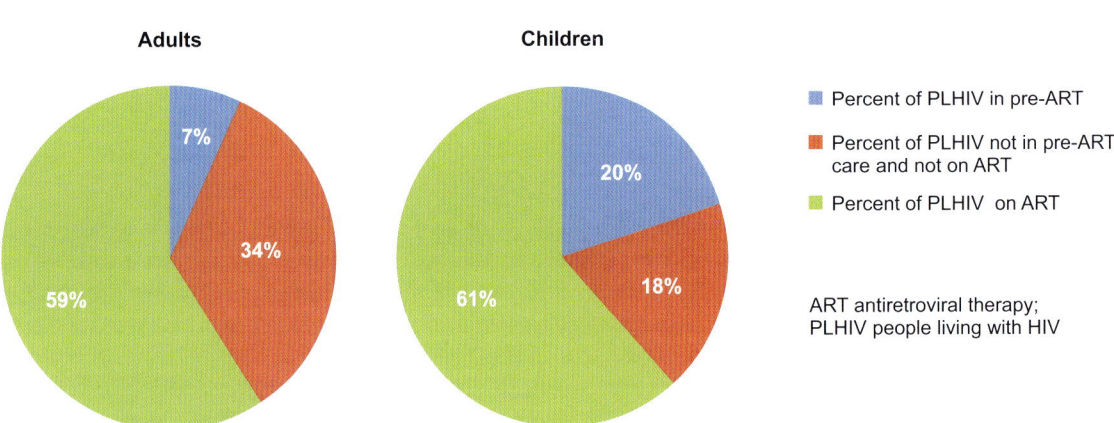

This scale-up was possible because of a CoC framework for delivery of comprehensive HIV services.[59,q] It built on the early involvement of peer support groups of people living with HIV called MMM[60] (Friends Help Friends Centres), and community-based care and support interventions.

Among the estimated total number of PLHIV, a significant proportion (34% in adults and 18% in children) is unaware of their HIV status or lost from HIV testing to enrollment into pre-ART care, or during pre-ART and ART. This indicates the need to further expand HTC coverage and to maximize linkages and retention throughout the processes from HTC, pre-ART and ART (Figures 11 and 13). Although HIV infection seems to be diagnosed earlier with HIV testing volumes increasing every year, most of the people living with HIV are seeking HIV testing and care only after they develop symptoms. The median CD4 count from 33 ART sites was 194 cells/μL (range of median counts across all sites: 76–496 cells/μL) in 2011, an increase from 112 cells/μL in 2006.[q] Other local studies show similar increases over time.[61] Review findings indicate that most new patients presenting at ART clinics are symptomatic and that the median CD4 counts at initial diagnosis and at the commencement of ART remain much lower than the recommended national CD4 count thresholds for

---

[q] National Center for HIV/AIDS, Dermatology and STDs, World Health Organization. Achievements and challenges of the continuum of care for PLHIV in Cambodia. Internal document. 2013.
[r] Poi Pet Health Centre ART/OI clinic: median CD4 at start of ART is 149 cells/μL (range 4–380 cells/μL), 3 May 2013.

ART initiation (<350 cells/μL).[r] It remains unclear why the CD4 count at start of treatment is so low if ART coverage at CD4 count <350 cells/μL is 81%. This should be investigated further and verified. A key question is why people are presenting late, and whether there is a selective drop-off in the cascade between testing, care and treatment, or whether current testing strategies are inadequate to find people relatively recently infected, or in fact whether this represents the dynamics of an "old" epidemic that peaked 15 years ago. It may be that the data presented are not accurate. In HIV-positive pregnant women and children, there is little information on the CD4 count at entry into services and at ART initiation.

Possible strategies to be considered for further improving the HIV treatment cascade are listed in Box 10.

Box 10: Improving the HIV treatment cascade

Some strategies worth considering to improve the HIV treatment cascade include:
(1) ensuring that symptomatic patients are staged clinically, using the WHO clinical staging, and started on ART while awaiting CD4 count results if at stages 3 and 4;
(2) tracking the appointments for regular CD4 monitoring in pre-ART patients and ensuring that they understand the importance of coming back if new symptoms occur;
(3) clinical triage to reduce waiting times in OI/ART clinics for very ill patients, pregnant women and young children;
(4) task-shifting or task-sharing following standardized protocols so that ART drug refills for stable and asymptomatic individuals can be provided by paramedical staff;
(5) accelerated protocols in counselling for treatment preparedness to reduce the three- to four-week delay in ART initiation for specific patients;
(6) community-level delivery of ART refill by peers; and
(7) spacing appointments for medical consultations such as three-monthly drug refills for patients who are stable on treatment and have a track record of adherence.

The proportion of people in pre-ART (~10%) is lower than that reported in other countries (30–50%) (Figure 13, HIV treatment cascade Cambodia, 2012). NCHADS reports indicate that there was high loss to follow-up and death during pre-ART care, although this has decreased from 35% in 2006 to 20% in 2011. However, the current reporting format and use of numbers in the quarterly and annual reports make it difficult to distinguish numerators and denominators, which is essential for understanding the proportion of loss during this stage. Pre-ART patients have higher attrition rates due to loss to follow up and death, compared to those already receiving ART. Of the 273 patients reported as lost to follow up in 2010–2011,[53] in fact 46.9% were lost to follow-up and 53.1% had died. Loss during the pre-ART stage represents a weakness in the care and support services. Thus, it would be important to characterize and understand the reasons for this high loss to follow up and death. Although modelling data indicate that mortality among people living with HIV has declined, there is a lack of information on causes of mortality in patients enrolled with the HIV services.[s] Scheduling regular care visits, active follow-up and treatment literacy education by health-care providers and nongovernmental organization/outreach personnel for those in pre-ART may prevent such attrition (see Box 10).

Cohort analysis of adults initiating treatment in 2006, 2009 and 2010 at 25, 31 and 34 OI/ART facilities, respectively, indicate that 93%, 84% and 78% of patients remained on ART after one, two and five years, respectively.[16] The 2012 HIV drug resistance EWI report[t] showed that nearly half (46% and 44%) of 46 adult and 27 paediatric OI/ART sites had issues with non-adherence to treatment, defined as <80% of all ART patients keeping their appointments. There is gradual attrition from ART care, and it is unclear what factors influence this loss. Factors affecting long-term adherence to ART, including pill-taking fatigue, need to be explored. In districts near the border of Thailand, migration for work (both adults and pregnant women)

---

[s] Vun MC. Trend on estimated death (modelling results), 2000–2015. From presentation on the Health sector response to HIV: progress made and way forward in Cambodia, 2013.
[t] Presentation on HIV drug resistance: early warning indicator study, 2012 (unpublished data).

seemed to be a major factor for loss to follow up from care. A common report noted during field visits was that HIV-positive persons on ART feel healthier and can go back to work. They migrate to Thailand for work and are lost from ART services in Cambodia; however, once symptomatic, they return home to access clinical care since there is no access to the publicly funded Thai health services for undocumented migrants. High out-of-pocket expenses, particularly for transport costs in rural areas due to the distance to ART sites at operational district level, and fragmented services are issues. The extent of treatment interruption as well as loss from the ART programme due to these factors is unknown and could not be assessed during the review.

There is a lack of data specific to key-affected populations, such as the proportion of entertainment workers, men who have sex with men, transgender persons and drug users who know their HIV status and access ART. These populations are estimated to account for around 40% of new HIV infections in the country.[17] Current voluntary counselling and testing and ART records could be adjusted to include information about these vulnerable populations. It is unclear as to what extent those who are HIV positive disclose their status and are offered additional peer support. As mentioned earlier, there is no "shared confidentiality" between the health services and the outreach/nongovernmental organization network. At present, outreach workers are not able to follow individuals through the HIV continuum of care and treatment cascade.

Paediatric HIV care (infants, children and adolescents)

In Cambodia, there is still a high infant mortality rate of 45 deaths per 1000 live births.[62,63] Forty per cent of all children below five years of age have chronic malnutrition (stunted), and 55% are anaemic. Children, particularly in rural areas and from poorer households, are more affected.[62] Because of weak maternal and child health services, care services for HIV-infected children including for HIV-exposed infants are also weak.

Children living with HIV are diagnosed late. Data from the National Paediatric Hospital in Phnom Penh show that two thirds of children admitted with known HIV status or at HIV diagnosis have a CD4 percentage of <25% and are in need of ART (see recommendations for HIV testing and counselling (personal communication, National Paediatric Hospital, Phnom Penh). The review team observed that "continuum of care for the family" is inadequate, from HIV testing to treatment for the family of HIV-positive parent(s) and their children. HIV-exposed infants are falling through the cracks because of the way services are organized. When women leave health facilities after delivery, they may not return for postpartum and newborn care at 6–8 weeks. There is no active follow-up system. Only half of the HIV-exposed infants have an early infant diagnosis at 6–8 weeks. Quality-of-care indicators for HIV-exposed infants, defined as the number "started on co-trimoxazole prophylaxis within two months of birth", show that only one third are receiving it.

Care for children living with HIV is complex as it encompasses multiple dimensions, and not just health and HIV. Children require chronic care and other support such as social welfare and education. Local studies note that children respond to and survive well with ART, and sociodemographic indicators such as being orphans may affect these outcomes.[64,65] Paediatric HIV care providers mentioned difficulties with appropriate disclosure of HIV status to the child. National Paediatric Hospital data showed that 60% of their cohort of HIV-infected children (N=1732) had lost one or both parents. Health-care providers reported difficulties in managing HIV-infected orphans and vulnerable children.

Review of available data from nongovernmental organizations supporting HIV-affected and -infected children suggest that in the next several years, there will be more HIV-infected children growing into adolescence and young adulthood. Of the 118 HIV-infected children under the care of a nongovernmental organization servicing rural populations, 61% were between 10 and 17 years of age (personal communication at site visit). Similarly, data from the National Paediatric Hospital indicate that two thirds of the 1752 HIV-infected children, half of whom are girls, are between 5 and 15 years of age. Health-care providers reported difficulties in transitioning HIV-positive adolescents to adult care. Adolescents, albeit having often been for many years with trusted paediatric care providers, will be referred to an unknown environment in adult care. Care for older children and adolescents needs to consider their developing sexuality, need for making sexual and reproductive health choices, and planning for life. Health-care workers reported that ensuring ART adherence in adolescents is difficult, particularly when the HIV status has not been disclosed to the adolescent.

Other issues reported during key informant interviews included stock-outs of paediatric drug formulations, necessitating the cutting of adult ART tablets. Treatment in young children under two years of age could not be adequately assessed. The involvement of MMM and nongovernmental organizations in home-based care activities for children could not be assessed. In Svay Rieng, the MMM group for adults included the adolescent child (who was infected through mother-to-child transmission) of one of the women living with HIV. The HIV-infected father had passed away.

There is an overall scarcity of data on paediatric HIV. These include information on transmission routes (presumably most are due to mother-to-child transmission), sex- and age-disaggregated analysis (by under two years, and two to five years of age), baseline CD4 count, treatment needs, sociodemographic indicators such as being orphaned, retention in pre-ART and ART care, including the spectrum of co-morbidities such as anaemia and malnutrition in HIV-infected infants and children.

Antiretroviral treatment guidelines

When to start

The 2012 national treatment guidelines[66] are in line with the 2010 WHO guidelines,[67] which recommend (i) starting ART at a CD4 count <350 cells/µL, (ii) starting TB therapy immediately after diagnosis of TB with co-trimoxazole prophylaxis, regardless of CD4 count, and starting ART immediately after two weeks of TB therapy, and (iii) triple ARV prophylaxis for pregnant women (Option B). The 2013 WHO consolidated guidelines for use of ARVs for treatment and prevention recommend starting ART at a CD4 count <500 cells/µL in adults and adolescents, regardless of clinical and immunological staging in pregnant women, serodiscordant couples, those with TB/HIV coinfection, hepatitis B/HIV coinfection and children under five years of age.[35]

In the context of high ART coverage, existing infrastructure, and the reported very small numbers not eligible for ART (10%), a move to start treatment at a CD4 count <500 cells/µL, including among key-affected populations, should be feasible with little additional investments.

A concept note on "treatment as prevention" was released by NCHADS in early 2013. This recommends treatment for the HIV-positive partner in serodiscordant couples at a CD4 count of 350–500 cells/µL and starting lifelong treatment for pregnant women, regardless of clinical and immunological staging. Serodiscordant couples account for 448 of 1210 estimated annual new HIV infections (Figure 14). With the few additional individuals and the low median CD4 count at enrolment, immediate ART for serodiscordant couples could be implemented at little additional investment for ARV drugs. As there is limited experience of the potential feasibility of targeting serodiscordant couples in concentrated epidemics with intensified prevention, documentation of the experience would help increase global knowledge. Moreover, Cambodia would be a good setting for considering "test and treat" in selected key-affected populations. There is an opportunity to develop demonstration projects to evaluate the acceptability and feasibility carefully in the Cambodian context, or to move more actively on this.

Figure 14: Modes of HIV transmission in Cambodia, 2013

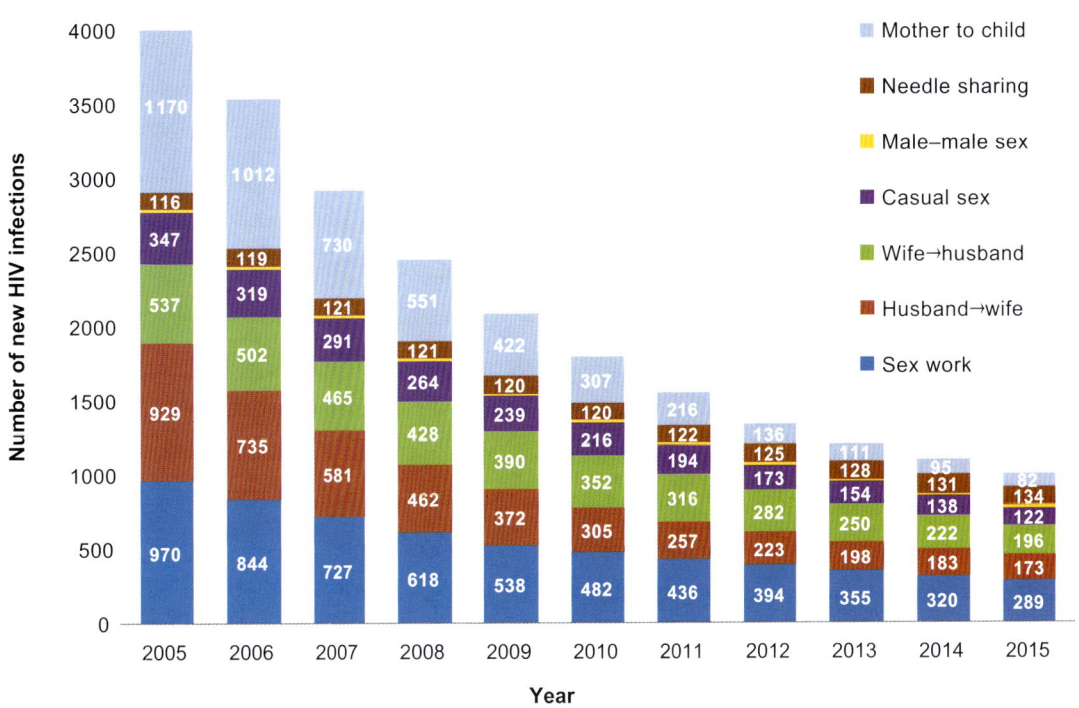

Source: Ministry of Health, National Center for HIV/AIDS, Dermatology and STDs. Estimations and projections of HIV/AIDS in Cambodia 2010–2015. Phnom Penh, Cambodia: 2011.

What to use

The 2012 national ART adult guideline continues to recommend stavudine (d4T) and lamivudine (3TC) as the preferred nucleoside reverse transcriptase inhibitors (NRTIs) in first-line regimens. The majority (52% and 79%) of adult and paediatric ART patients received d4T regimens in 2011. The 2010 and 2013 WHO guidelines recommend the use of tenofovir disoproxil fumarate (TDF)-based regimens plus a non-nucleoside reverse transcriptase inhibitor (NNRTI) and phasing out of d4T. For pregnant women, the 2011 national guidelines on PMTCT recommend zidovudine (AZT)-based regimens in line with the WHO 2010 guidelines. However, the 2013 WHO guidelines promote harmonization of PMTCT regimens with adult regimens.

In the process of aligning with WHO guidelines, a transition plan has been drafted by NCHADS to move towards using TDF-based regimens for adult treatment, including initiating all new patients (and pregnant women) on TDF-based regimens, and shifting those currently taking d4T to TDF. Challenges will include ensuring adequate procurement and supply of TDF in 2013–2014, and appropriate clinical assessment for treatment failure before changing to the TDF/3TC/efavirenz (EFV) once-a-day combination. A draft transition plan[u] to TDF requires all patients to test for creatinine clearance and/or serum phosphate, which may increase out-of-pocket expenses for the patient if this test is not free within the health services. The transition plan should be reviewed and updated in line with the WHO 2013 guidelines and also for the use of TDF in children and adolescents. Another challenge will be the transition from d4T-based regimens to AZT in children in the context of a high background prevalence of childhood anaemia.

---

[u] Internal NCHADS document under development. Available on request from NCHADS.

Current second-line regimens include lopinavir/ritonavir (LPV/r) combined with two other drugs such as didanosine (ddI), AZT, 3TC or TDF. Protease inhibitor-based regimens were administered to about 4% of adults and 8.5% of children in 2011,[53] a slight increase from 3.8% and 7.2%, respectively, in 2010.[68] A study of 70 patients receiving second-line regimens showed that most (92.3%) had undetectable viral load at 24 months of follow up, indicating that the current second-line regimen is effective.[69]

There are indications that third-line regimens and drugs may be required in the near future. In a recent study of 89 patients experiencing virological failure (viral load >250 copies/mL) after at least six months on an LPV/r-based second-line regimen, one third (29/89) required switching to a third-line regimen.[70] Further guidance in this area relies on expert opinion.

MMM (self-help group) and home-based care

"Shared care" between the health services and the MMM/nongovernmental home-based care network seemed not to be functioning optimally. In most sites visited, newly diagnosed HIV-infected individuals were referred to the ART counsellor. In Svay Rieng referral hospital, it was reported that patients with positive test results were referred to the self-help group MMM for counselling and referral to pre-ART and ART services. However, when the review team met with MMM, the group did not appear to be functioning effectively. Group meetings had only occurred once or twice during the past year. In Banteay Meanchey province, MMM volunteers were located within the ART/pre-ART clinics and were providing essential additional support to clinic activities, including registration of patients, peer counselling, tracking of defaulters and coordination with local nongovernmental organizations and peer networks. The review noted that the MMM scheme, for which standard operating procedures were developed in 2006, had evolved and was functional in some sites but not in others. In provinces where there is active donor and partner support such as in Battambang and Banteay Meanchey, the network seemed to function more cohesively with the health services. Key informants reported that there are regular coordination problems between health staff and the MMM/nongovernmental home-based care, where the roles and responsibilities of the peer network are not clearly articulated within the pre-ART/ART health services. This scheme will require a comprehensive review and strong coordination at all levels to fit into the current needs of the national programme and the Cambodia 3.0 strategy.

Discussions during the field visits with nongovernmental organization and outreach workers indicate that outreach following the standard operating procedures for home-based care is being delivered to individuals and families (adults, pregnant women and families, including orphans and vulnerable children). For the volunteers interviewed, there is high satisfaction with the support given, which ranges from transport and incidental cash support, peer counselling, treatment education and family support, including for orphans and vulnerable children. A nongovernmental organization in Banteay Meanchey had provided technical and seed funding to support micro-financing and livelihood initiatives of peer-led groups of people living with HIV. Overall, the care and support activities, including cash reimbursement for transport, contributed to utilization of HIV and ART services, particularly for rural populations; children living with HIV received care at a tertiary paediatric pre-ART/ART site.

Other care and support

The national sexual and reproductive health strategy for 2006–2010[71] does not include specific recommendations for counselling on reproductive choices and family planning for HIV-positive women. Observations during field visits suggest that only some health centres offer family planning, including for HIV-positive women. The strategy recommends integration of HIV testing in other sexual and reproductive health services, including family planning.

Co-morbidities not related to HIV (diabetes, hypertension, dyslipidaemia, etc.), which will occur due to an ageing adult cohort, are not well understood in the Cambodian context. The increasing use of protease inhibitors may result in such co-morbidities among people living with HIV and should be assessed.

Recommendations

5.6 Ongoing efforts to update the 2012 national ART guidelines and the 2012 concept note on "treatment as prevention" in line with the new 2013 WHO guidelines should continue. An evaluation after one year of the change in threshold for starting ART and ability to implement that change, as well as the effect on median CD4 count at start of ART, would help inform Cambodia 3.0 (*see* Box 11). Increasing access to ART for key-affected populations is an immediate priority.

5.7 Ongoing efforts to phase out d4T and introduce TDF for adults, adolescents and children should continue. Ensuring appropriate and adequate procurement and supply of TDF and paediatric formulations to treat the range of age- and weight-band groups according to guidelines is an important improvement in HIV care for adults and children.

5.8 NCHADS may consider improving the existing mechanisms to support and promote adherence and retention, and minimize loss to follow up through task-sharing as a part of decentralization of treatment. This could include a review of the current scheme with MMM and enhancing coordination at all levels to fit into the current needs of the national programme and the 3.0 strategy. For example, active case management could be done by trained people living with HIV, drawn from health centres, MMM groups of people living with HIV or peer outreach workers, and the role of ART counsellors expanded to serve as case managers to help staff at the ART clinics. This would strengthen the interface between facility, community and home-based care.

5.9 Strengthening institutional capacity would be important for providing paediatric and adolescent HIV care, including age-appropriate disclosure of HIV status to the child and adolescent, addressing emerging sexuality needs during adolescence and young adulthood, as well as transitioning to adult services. Renewed focus on the "family continuum of care" would support the 3.0 strategy.

5.10 It is suggested that further assessment of paediatric and adolescent HIV care and treatment, including for HIV-exposed infants, incorporate an analysis of the data from various cohorts to understand the quality of paediatric and adolescent care services, and whether current recording and reporting systems are equipped to provide data useful for the programme.

5.11 Linking NCHADS with maternal and child health services is advised for offering other care services, including sexual and reproductive health, family planning and cervical cancer screening for women living with HIV and female entertainment workers. Emerging co-morbidities from noncommunicable diseases due to the prolonged provision of ART may also be considered.

Box 11: Anticipating adaptation of monitoring systems in line with the 2013 WHO guidelines

The changing guidelines imply a review and update of the ART initiation form for adults to see if it is capturing reasons for delayed testing and referral, and transmission risks to get better information on patients newly starting ART, and to be able to monitor trends over time. The forms should ensure that pregnant women are clearly identified and their data analysable in the ART database. While there is a variable for this in the current monitoring forms, the information and the patients are not captured well. The database should be able to see and analyse the number of pregnant women already on ART, those newly identified and starting B+ for PMTCT.

Prevention of mother-to-child transmission (PMTCT) of HIV

The National Maternal and Child Health Center (NMCHC) oversees infant, child, adolescent and maternal health under several components, such as nutrition, Expanded Programme on Immunization, sexual and reproductive health including cervical cancer prevention, and infant and young child feeding. Integration of HIV interventions with maternal and child health services to enable and sustain HIV testing and provision of ARVs for HIV-infected women, including pregnant women and children, will be important. The NMCHC is in charge of the national PMTCT programme.

Cambodia has achieved universal coverage of treatment needs and is well poised to pioneer "B+", which entails offering immediate ART to all pregnant women in a low-prevalence, concentrated epidemic setting,[35] but challenges remain. There has been rapid expansion of coverage of PMTCT programmes, saturating almost all 1061 maternal and child health services. In 2012, of the 377 340 estimated pregnancies, most (99%) pregnant women attended antenatal care at least once. Of these, 89% received HIV testing, although only 82% received their test results: 1153 (0.3%) were found to be HIV-infected and 65.1% of them received ARVs during pregnancy and/or delivery (Table 4). However, only 73% of HIV-exposed infants received ARV prophylaxis for the first six weeks to reduce mother-to-child transmission. Of the exposed infants, 33.2% had early infant testing (in the first several months of life), with low rates of early positive test results but high rates of loss to follow up. Data on outcomes of early infant diagnosis, and treatment for HIV-exposed infants and those who tested HIV positive, are not available.

Syphilis testing is currently not routinely offered in antenatal care, although available data indicate that maternal syphilis rates are low (Table 3).

The review team found that there is a discrepancy in the data collected by the HIV and maternal and child health programmes for various indicators and reported in various documents. This seems to result from different systems being used by each programme for recording and reporting, and the lack of common patient identifiers across programmes. Table 4 gives data consolidated from the global AIDS reporting submitted in April 2013 to WHO and UNAIDS. With the high attrition along the care cascade for PMTCT, modelled data from 2012 suggest an overall national mother-to-child transmission rate of 10%.

Currently, the Cambodia target is to lower the transmission rate to 5% by 2015 and 2% by 2020. Specific data on the outcomes of infants, children and adolescents are unavailable. Determinants influencing loss from the care cascade need investigation. Strengthening the continuum of care and improving longitudinal monitoring and assessing impact will be even more important as Cambodia moves to the B+ approach of providing ART to all pregnant and breastfeeding women with HIV.

Little is known about provision of ART and PMTCT services by the private sector. If Cambodia aspires to reach virtual elimination, it will be important to undertake a situation analysis to review the potential of using the private sector to provide ARVs for PMTCT and examine how this can be integrated with the national programme.

Opportunities to integrate HIV into interventions that comprehensively address the pregnancy–infant–early childhood care continuum such as the "1000 days" nutrition campaign could be valuable to improve breastfeeding practices for HIV-infected babies. Informal review of data suggests that 50% or more of HIV-exposed infants are being partially or fully formula fed, in part due to prior recommendations and training on formula feeding. Moving to Option B+ provides an opportunity to strengthen messaging and support for exclusive breastfeeding of HIV-exposed infants for the first six months of life and appropriate young child feeding according to the national guidelines.

Integrated follow up of exposed infants by the Expanded Programme on Immunization, including the newly adopted second dose of measles immunization at 18–24 months of age, should be implemented in both the immunization outpatient clinic and the paediatric ART clinic (for early infant diagnosis and further care). Clinical assessment and HIV antibody testing of HIV exposed infants could occur at that visit.

Follow up of mother–baby pairs in the PMTCT cascade is the major priority for the maternal and child health and HIV programmes. Maternal and child health reporting systems for PMTCT at the national, provincial and district levels are linked to the Cambodian HMIS, which are web-based and online. Data are reported monthly from antenatal services and transmitted on paper to the district office, which enters the information into the electronic database. Individual information on mother–baby pairs is available to allow longitudinal tracking of outcomes up to the 18-month confirmatory HIV test (Figure 16). Since 2009, in order to consolidate a holistic picture of women entering care for PMTCT and mother–baby outcomes, follow up using the PMTCT tree allows detailed reporting of the cascade by operational districts and at national level, linked to the HMIS for maternal and child health. Currently, 22 operational districts in eight provinces provide reports as training is being expanded to cover all districts in 2013.

Figure 15: Example of tracking the PMTCT cascade through the "PMTCT tree" in Banteay Meanchey province

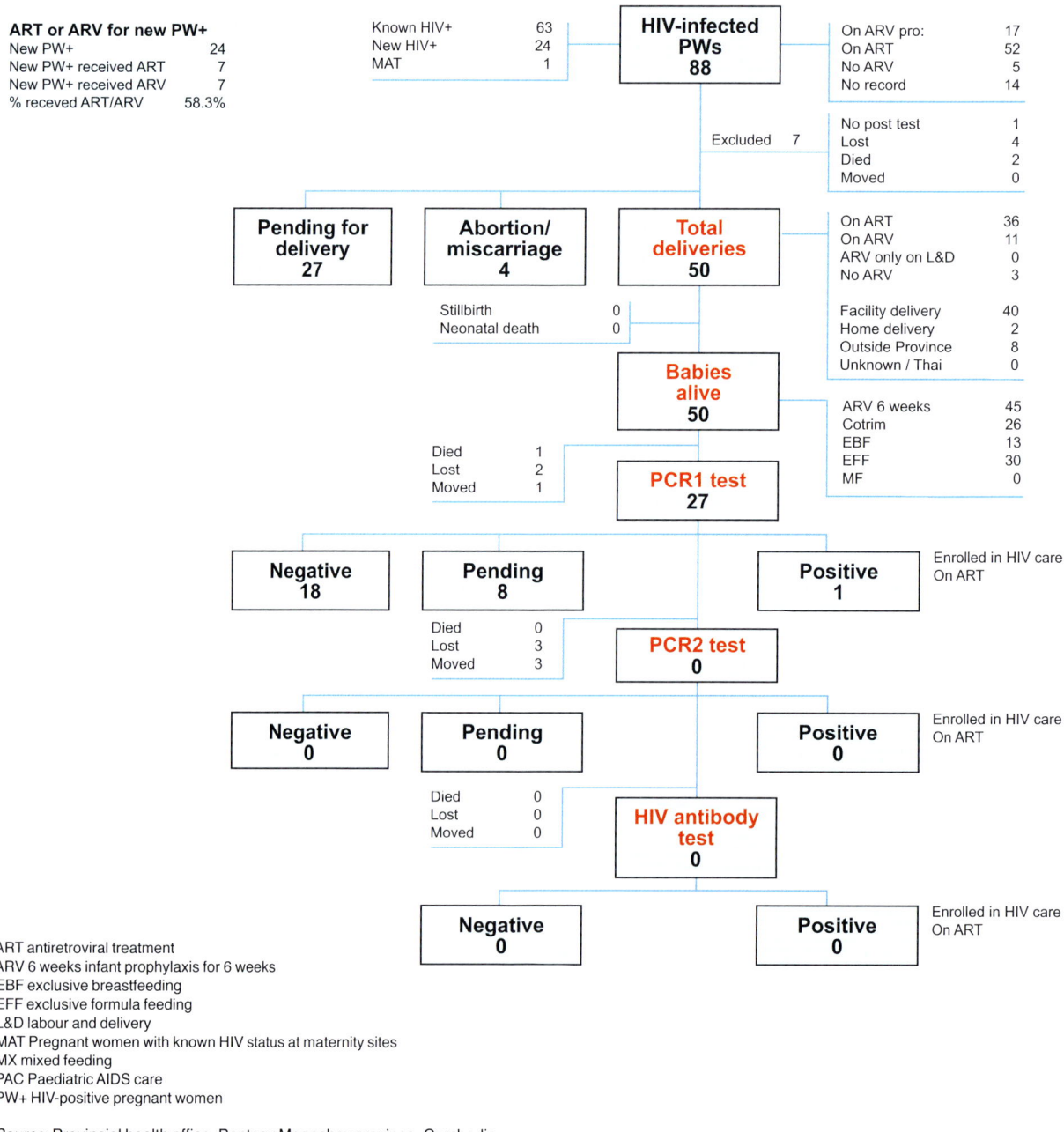

ART antiretroviral treatment
ARV 6 weeks infant prophylaxis for 6 weeks
EBF exclusive breastfeeding
EFF exclusive formula feeding
L&D labour and delivery
MAT Pregnant women with known HIV status at maternity sites
MX mixed feeding
PAC Paediatric AIDS care
PW+ HIV-positive pregnant women

Source: Provincial health office, Banteay Meanchey province, Cambodia

Recommendations

5.12 The standard operating procedures for the Boosted Linked Response by both NMCHC and NCHADS support PMTCT Option B+. It is recommended that implementation of these standard operating procedures be actively pursued (*see* Box 12), and the relevant documents disseminated to district and health centre levels (not just at the provincial level).

5.13 NCHADS and NMCHC should develop clear targets for both coverage and final outcome measures for 2015. It would also be necessary to calculate annual mother-to-child transmission rates based on the cohort data from PMTCT programmes and infant outcomes through 2020, for both ART and maternal and child health.

5.14 The PMTCT programme may consider a routine offer of combined screening for haemoglobin, HIV, syphilis and hepatitis testing to pregnant women attending antenatal care, as part of basic antenatal screening, and monitor its uptake.

5.15 It is suggested that enhanced linkages among the current data systems of the maternal and child health programme and NCHADS be established so that subset analysis could be performed for the needs of each programme, e.g. ART in pregnant women and infants/children/adolescents.

5.16 A situation analysis may be considered to review private sector involvement in HIV services.

Box 12: Option B+ for PMTCT and interlinked patient monitoring systems

As Cambodia moves to adopt Option B+, active monitoring and reporting on the progress and limitations of the approach are necessary, particularly on the adherence to and retention of women on lifelong treatment. Establishing the final status of infection and health outcomes in the child are equally important.

Patient information systems need to be adapted towards longitudinal follow up to allow evaluation of outcomes for Option B+. This will require an interlinked patient monitoring system, which allows identification of pregnant women in existing ART cohorts, in addition to unique health identifiers.

Monitoring the cascade

Despite these challenges, Cambodia is well positioned to implement the 3.0 strategy designed to address elimination of new HIV infections in a low-prevalence, concentrated epidemic setting. This will require improved coordination and integrated management of the HIV testing and care cascades for adults, pregnant women and children by both NCHADS and NMCHC. Programmatic flexibility to adapt and sustain service delivery models, including innovations to support active case management and outreach at the community level, would be required to optimize retention. There is a culture of documentation and reporting within the health services which can be used to good advantage. Systems are in place at a number of pre-ART/ART sites to periodically review and follow up indicators on programme quality and outcomes, for example, through the CQI. Sustaining these systems and increasing their coverage will be essential for maintaining and improving the quality of services, particularly as services continue to evolve. Strengthening data systems through linkages and integration of formats, and adapting towards longitudinal follow up by NCHADS and NMCHC will allow for better assessment of infant infections, maternal health, child, adolescent and adult survival, and loss along the cascade of services.

Table 4: Prevention of mother-to-child transmission data, 2012

Indicator	Proportion (numerator/denominator)
% of pregnant women attending antenatal care at least once during the reporting period	99.2% (374 986/377 340)
% of pregnant women attending antenatal care at least once during the reporting period and who were tested	89.4% (337 528/377 340)
% of pregnant women who were tested for HIV and received their results – during pregnancy, during labour and delivery, and during the postpartum period (<72 hours), including those with previously known HIV status	81.7% (308 245/377 340)
% of pregnant women who were tested for HIV and received their results with positive HIV test result (including those previously known to be positive)	0.3% (1153/337 528)
% of pregnant women with known HIV infection attending antenatal care for a new pregnancy	49.3% (569/1153)
% of pregnant women attending antenatal care whose male partner was tested for HIV in the past 12 months	17.0% (65 491/374 986)
% of HIV-positive pregnant women who received ARVs to reduce the risk of mother-to-child transmission during pregnancy and delivery	65.1% (862/1324)
– which is lifelong ART	84.1% (725/862)
– maternal Option B	11.8% (102/862)
– maternal Option A	4.1% (35/862)
% of infants born to HIV-infected women (HIV-exposed infants) who received ARV prophylaxis to reduce the risk of early mother-to-child-transmission in the first 6 weeks (i.e. early postpartum transmission around 6 weeks of age)	72.5% (960/1324)
% of infants born to HIV-infected women (HIV-exposed infants) who were provided with ARVs (either mother or infant) to reduce the risk of HIV transmission during the breastfeeding period	No data

Source: Cambodia global AIDS reporting 2013 (Ref: Excel sheets final consolidated, 4 April 2013)

Increasing the use of routine programme data will be essential for assessing programme performance and evaluating key areas under field conditions. This would include data from the new 3.0 HIV testing procedures, STI testing, service delivery models (boosted linked response), and new policies and concepts such as Option B+, earlier treatment and treatment regardless of clinical and immunological staging. Such data would also be needed for understanding factors that may reduce efficiency and for developing strategies to improve the programme.

Recommendations

5.17 Regular use is recommended of different types of data including routine programme data to understand the patient cohort and provide data for decision-making, assess programme performance and address bottlenecks along the cascades at national and subnational levels.

5.18 Impact analysis and evaluation of outcomes could be strengthened, as they are critical to inform whether algorithms and interventions are working.

6. Tuberculosis and HIV

In 2012, CENAT reported 40 258 newly registered TB patients; in addition, 4.4% (1423) of the 32 359 who were tested for HIV had a positive test result (Figure 16). The 2012 WHO global TB report[72] shows that the estimated TB prevalence of 817/100 000 population and TB mortality rates of 63/100 000 are among the highest in the 22 high-burden countries globally. The second TB prevalence survey in 2011 showed a remarkable 45% reduction in bacteriologically confirmed cases compared to 2002. The HIV prevalence among TB patients declined from 13% in 2009 to 4.4% in 2012, a threefold decrease. In August 2012, a joint TB programme review facilitated by WHO and partners was conducted. The report was reviewed and HIV/TB related findings updated by the HIV review team.[7]

TB/HIV is well integrated within the services for directly observed treatment, short-course for TB (DOTS) and CoC framework in operational districts (Table 5). Although paper based, the TB monitoring system produces reliable data for the programme. Current coverage is high for routine HIV testing (85%), co-trimoxazole prophylaxis (99%) and ART (89%) among newly registered TB patients. The proportion of TB/HIV coinfected individuals starting ART has increased from 14% in 2009 to 89% in 2012, a remarkable sixfold increase. Screening for TB among people living with HIV was 85% in 2012; of the 3411 screened, 27% had active TB.[7]

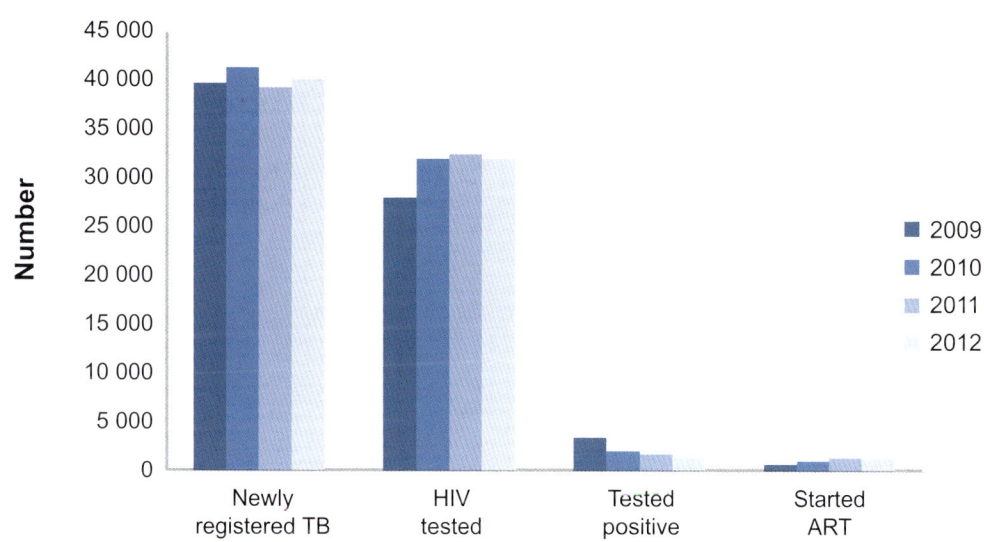

Figure 16: TB/HIV: From diagnosis to treatment, 2009–2012

The current TB monitoring system does capture most of this information among TB patients, whereas NCHADS is supposed to capture information on TB/HIV coinfected individuals once they complete TB treatment and are transferred to ART services. The *Three I's for HIV/TB* – infection control, intensified TB case-finding and isoniazid preventive therapy – are implemented (Table 6).[73] Active TB cases are treated in TB treatment centres. Less than 60% of pre-ART/ART sites (35 out of 61) currently provide isoniazid preventive therapy. It is estimated that, at present, less than one quarter of screened people living with HIV receive isoniazid preventive therapy. TB deaths among people living with HIV are not recorded.

This review team confirmed the findings of the joint TB programme review[7]; that there seems to be a discrepancy in the data collected by the TB and HIV programmes for various indicators. This seems to result from different systems being used by each programme for recording and reporting, and the lack of common patient identifiers across programmes.

Table 5: TB and HIV services in Cambodia (by March 2013)

TB services

- TB diagnostic facilities: 1200
- TB microscopy centres: 214
- TB culture laboratories: 3 (including one doing DST of first line drugs)
- Xpert® MTB/RIF
- TB treatment available from 1071 health facilities

HIV services

- PITC for pregnant women and TB cases: more than 1000
- Voluntary counselling and testing centres: 253
- CD4 laboratories: 6 regional labs, 3 in Phnom Penh
- Pre-ART/ART centres: 61 in 50 operational districts and 21 provinces and cities*
- Pre-ART/ART centres implementing *Three I's* (mainly IPT): 37, out of which 3 are using tuberculin skin testing for IPT

DST drug-susceptibility testing; IPT isoniazid preventive therapy; PITC provider-initiated testing and counselling
Source: Third quarterly comprehensive report, 2012. HIV/AIDS prevention and care programme, Ministry of Health, National Center for AIDS, Dermatology and STDs (NCHADS website)

Table 6: Performance of TB/HIV collaborative activities at national level, by year, 2009–2012

Indicators	2009	2010	2011	2012
No. (%) of new adult PLHIV screened for TB (a)	4667/7071 (66%)	3598/5104 (70%)	4757/5596 (85%)	3411
Of (a), no. (%) found to have TB (b)	1539 (33%)	1110 (31%)	1187 (22%)	918 (27%)
Of (b), no. started on anti-TB treatment*	NA	NA	NA	NA
Of (a), no. started on IPT	43	188	1043	944
No. (%) of TB patients tested for HIV (c)	28 246/40 199 (70%)	32 236/41 628 (77%)	32 544/39 670 (82%)	32 359/40 258 (80%)
Of (c), no. (%) found HIV- positive (d)	3597 (13%)	2112 (6.6%)	1650 (5.1%)	1423 (4.4%)
Of (d), no. (%) started/continued on CPT	1081 (30%)	1383 (65%)	1456 (88%)	1410 (99%)
Of (d), no. (%) started/continued on ART	526 (14%)	944 (45%)	1306 (79%)	1268 (89%)

ART antiretroviral therapy; CPT co-trimoxazole preventive therapy; IPT isoniazid preventive therapy; PLHIV people living with HIV
* The current NCHADS data system does not capture this information. Active TB cases are treated in TB treatment centres.

Active TB case detection in closed settings has started. In Svay Rieng provincial prison, evaluation team members observed a mobile team conducting clinical screening, and suspected cases undergoing chest X-ray, sputum smear and Xpert MTB/RIF testing. However, HIV testing was not offered. The review team observed that there was no implementation of isoniazid preventive therapy for people living with HIV and TB infection, and that there were no TB infection control measures in the Svay Rieng provincial prison.

Recommendations

6.1 The HIV review team endorses the recommendations on TB/HIV made by the Joint TB programme review in 2012[7] and their implementation (*see* action points in Box 13).

6.2 Efforts to reduce TB deaths among people living with HIV will require enhanced efforts not only for HIV case detection and provision of co-trimoxazole prophylaxis and ART, but also for active case detection of TB, and provision of isoniazid preventive therapy and TB treatment among people living with HIV.

6.3 Current efforts at active TB case-finding in closed settings should be complemented by the systematic offer of HIV testing and further expansion of TB infection control measures.

6.4 Establishing a corresponding computerized electronic TB programme database could help in the harmonization of data collection, validation and analysis at all levels of services across the two programmes.

6.5 It is advised that TB diagnosis among people living with HIV using Xpert MTB/RIF be expanded nationwide as soon as possible.

Box 13: Recommendations on TB/HIV made by the joint TB programme review in 2012[7]

(1) Implementation of the *Three I's* (mainly isoniazid preventive therapy) in all pre-ART/ART sites could be expanded by:
    (a) ensuring that the HIV programme train staff in new pre-ART/ART sites on the *Three I's*; and
    (b) providing isoniazid preventive therapy to new pre-ART/ART sites through the TB programme.

(2) Staff of both programmes in each operational district could strengthen the feedback mechanism and meet at least once a month to exchange data. By defining the responsibilities for reporting on different indicators, the quality of reporting would improve. CENAT and NCHADS would need to provide support for this.

(3) It is suggested that NCHADS consider changing the indicator and increase the activity to report all (new and old) people living with HIV screened for TB in any reporting period.

(4) According to WHO recommendations,[73] tuberculin skin testing is not a requirement for initiating isoniazid preventive therapy. Hence, programmes may consider giving isoniazid preventive therapy to all people living with HIV with no symptoms suggestive of TB, including those who are on ART.

(5) It is recommended that referral and feedback mechanisms between both programmes be strengthened:
    (a) At the regional hospital level, more frequent meetings could be held between TB and HIV programme staff (preferably weekly) to exchange data on referral.
    (b) At the operational district level, referral and feedback could be discussed by TB and HIV staff at least on a monthly basis. A case-management approach might be considered to strengthen efficiency. Quarterly review meetings could also be utilized to strengthen this mechanism.
    (c) Regular communication is suggested between health centre staff and pre-ART/ART staff for feedback on referrals, especially on TB treatment initiation.

(6) *See* the section on "Supervision, monitoring and evaluation" [of the joint TB review report] for the recommendation on electronic TB programme data.

7. HIV/STI laboratory services

HIV and STI laboratory services, such as HIV rapid testing, syphilis testing, CD4 count, early infant diagnosis and viral load testing, are established and available within the health services (Table 7). National reference laboratories are located at NCHADS and the National Institute of Public Health with an established division of roles and responsibilities. The NCHADS laboratory was set up in 2011 with US Government and other donor support as a centralized model to provide high-quality and rapid turnaround for CD4 testing, viral load and drug resistance services to hospitals and ART facilities in the Phnom Penh area and nationwide. The laboratory staff is also responsible for building capacity and overseeing HIV and STI laboratory services throughout the country. The National Institute of Public Health serves as the public health reference laboratory responsible for the external quality assurance system (EQAS)[74] for HIV antibody tests and early infant diagnosis.

Both laboratories perform CD4 counts for different hospitals in defined coverage areas. The US CDC provides continued technical support in this area. Nearly all the costs of running the HIV and STI laboratories (reagents, commodities, consumables) are supported by the Global Fund, with smaller contributions for specific activities from partners such as US CDC, WHO, United Nations Children's Fund (UNICEF) and Clinton Health Access Initiative (CHAI). Current issues include high workload at NCHADS with the present staffing levels, inadequate periodic laboratory supervision and assessment at provincial services.

The NCHADS laboratory is responsible for STI quality assurance. However, apart from screening for syphilis (using rapid plasma reagin/ Venereal Disease Research Laboratory [RPR/VDRL] and *Treponema pallidum* haemagglutination assay [TPHA], and cervicitis (by Gram stain), there is little etiological diagnosis of STI and monitoring in the programme, as the national STI protocol uses syndromic management. Gonorrhoea antimicrobial resistance surveillance has not been regularly done by the programme.

Table 7: Availability of HIV and STI tests

Level of laboratories	HIV and STI tests available	Role
National reference laboratory: NCHADS	ELISA, viral load, CD4 RPR/VDRL, TPHA, Gram stain, real-time PCR for gonorrhoea and chlamydia	EQAS, quality control for STI surveillance, viral load monitoring
National reference laboratory: National Institute of Public Health	CD4, DNA PCR, Western Blot for HIV-1 and -2	EQAS (VCT), early infant diagnosis, research
Referral hospital (provincial and operational district level)	HIV, RPR/VDRL, TPHA, Gram stain, CD4 (a few hospitals)	Service[a], viral load specimen linkage to apex labs[b]
Health centre	RPR/VDRL, TPHA (selected), HIV[d]	Service

ELISA enzyme-linked immunosorbent assay; EQAS external quality assurance system; PCR polymerase chain reaction; RPR rapid plasma reagin; STI sexually transmitted infection; TPHA *Treponema pallidum* haemagglutination assay; VCT voluntary counselling and testing; VDRL Venereal Disease Research Laboratory
[a] Where pre-ART/ART clinics for paediatric HIV are located, transportation for dried blood spot is available.
[b] Viral load blood specimens are sent by primary care systems to the provincial laboratory.
[c] ELISA and rapid tests
[d] Rapid test

Quality assurance systems are established for HIV testing at voluntary counselling and testing sites. The National Institute of Public Health has conducted EQAS for voluntary counselling and testing sites that have been functioning for at least six months (217 out of 253 in 2012). Similarly, EQAS for the nine FACSCounts available in the country for estimating CD4 counts is being conducted regularly with the involvement of the six machines in provincial hospitals and three in Phnom Penh (two NCHADS, one National Institute of Public Health). In the future, the programme plans to procure 10 point-of-care CD4 count machines (PIMA™).[v]

Viral load testing using the Abbott automated molecular diagnostics system, the m2000 platform, is available at NCHADS. Blood specimen transport systems from pre-ART/ART sites are established. Table 8 shows past results. A second viral load laboratory is planned in Battambang. The throughputs of the NCHADS laboratory for viral load should be higher than 100 per week. Depending on the number of samples coming in, the machine can be run almost every day, and it is usually run at least 2–3 times a week (up to 96 samples per run).

Current unit cost per viral load test is approximately US$ 25 per test, which is high if the programme is to use viral load routinely for monitoring patients on ART. As the use of viral load monitoring increases, this may be limited by current capacities (availability of machines and staff) and high unit cost of the test.

Early infant diagnosis using the Roche DNA PCR Amplicor 1.5 was established at the end of 2007 at the National Institute of Public Health laboratory. About 1000 tests are done annually, linked to 35 paediatric pre-ART/ART sites nationwide. A reagent stock-out since May 2013 has been reported. The National Institute of Public Health, with the support of US CDC, will be introducing an electronic database system for early infant diagnosis data in 2013. This will streamline the process of linking results to the original specimen identifiers provided by the referring facilities in the provinces. Efforts are under way to streamline management and implementation of virological testing and increase testing volumes on the Abbott device with the support of CHAI.

HIV drug-resistance testing is not available in Cambodia. Currently, samples for HIV drug resistance testing are collected for research or for HIV drug resistance surveillance activities. Samples are collected and sent to the China Center for Disease Control and Prevention for sequencing, with funding support from WHO Cambodia.

Table 8: Viral load test results, 25/04/2011 till 18/02/2013

Viral load (copies/ml)	Number (total N=9402)	Percentage (%)
Undetected	6377	67.8
<50	1298	13.8
50–1000	483	5.2
>1000	1244	13.2

Note: 47.6% were women. Age range: 1–79 years (239 [2.5%] were 1–4 years; 3088 [32.8%] were 5–15 years of age; however, there were missing/corrupted data in this field). Current laboratory request formats do not indicate ART/clinical data and these data are not linked to the ART database; thus there is limited use of these data to determine the proportion of patients with ART failure.

---

[v] This type of CD4 analyser enables CD4 T-cell analysis at the point of care from a finger-stick or venous whole blood sample in 20 minutes.

The database for early infant diagnosis collects information on HIV-exposed infants tested and their test results. It was reported to the review team that there were instances in the provinces when the laboratory was not able to report test results to the clinic. The team was told that there is no consistent system to link test results to the mother–baby pairs who participate in the PMTCT programme.

Recommendations

7.1 In order to oversee, supervise, build capacity and monitor overall HIV/STI laboratory capacities, it is recommended that national reference laboratories be strengthened. Enhancing the laboratories would entail the strengthening of human resources, technology and coordination between apex services. It is suggested that the patient information systems on early infant diagnosis be strengthened so that the records of mother and infant pairs are linked. Ideally, the early infant diagnosis database would be linked to the patient monitoring database of NCHADS and PMTCT.

7.2 As recommended in the 2013 WHO treatment guidelines, NCHADS should consider investing more in viral load monitoring, and set reasonable goals for 2015 and 2020 to allow appropriate planning for resource needs. Engaging with partners would help NCHADS to think about how best to utilize CD4 counts in a changing environment.

7.3 It is recommended that coverage of the EQAS programmes for HIV and STI antibody testing be sustained and cover the full array of tests in all facilities providing HIV testing. These would include HIV and syphilis rapid tests, validation of HIV testing algorithms using rapid tests, CD4 count and viral load, as well as early infant diagnosis.

7.4 Innovative diagnostic approaches, including point-of-care CD4 counts, and point-of-care molecular diagnostic platforms such as GeneXpert® for HIV viral load, chlamydia and gonorrhoea may be considered.

7.5 It is advised that existing STI surveillance be strengthened with periodic etiological studies and gonococcal antimicrobial resistance monitoring (GASP) to support STI case management.

8. Pharmaceutical supply management

Product financing

The main pharmaceutical and health product groups related to HIV/AIDS in Cambodia are ARV drugs, laboratory diagnostics and reagents, drugs to treat OI/STI, and blood safety commodities (Table 9).

ARV drugs used in the public health programmes of Cambodia are entirely financed by the Global Fund through the principal recipient NCHADS. HIV diagnostics and laboratory reagents are also entirely financed by the Global Fund via NCHADS. Current forecasts and procurement plans submitted to and approved by the Global Fund show that around US$ 3.5 million worth of laboratory supplies will be needed per year. OI and STI medicines provided by NCHADS to the ART sites are funded by the Global Fund (around US$ 350 000 per year). Blood safety products (blood bags, blood tests, gloves, etc.) used by the national blood bank system are almost entirely financed by the Government of Cambodia.

Table 9: Source(s) of funding, responsibility for forecasting, procurement and storage/distribution of medical supplies, by type of health product groups, Cambodia, 2013

	US$ funding	National forecasting	Procurement	Storage and distribution
Antiretroviral drugs	100% Global Fund US$ 5.5 M/year	NCHADS Forecasting Working Group and Logistics Management Unit with assistance from CHAI	Voluntary pooled procurement[a]	Central Medical Store
Laboratory diagnostics and reagents	100% Global Fund US$ 3.5 M/year	NCHADS Forecasting Working Group (but not clear who/how/when)		
Drugs to treat opportunistic and sexually transmitted infections	Global Fund US$ 0.3 M/year Government	NCHADS Forecasting Working Group and Logistics Management Unit using consumption-based quantification tool developed by WHO officer based at Department of Drugs and Food but no clear system		
Blood safety	Government	National Blood Transfusion Centre	Government	National Blood Transfusion Centre

[a] The voluntary pooled procurement mechanism has been established by the Global Fund to assist countries with insufficient international procurement capacity or which require rather small product volumes.
Source: NCHADS Logistics Management Unit

Product selection

Cambodia's national guidelines for ART in adults and adolescents were updated in 2012 based on the 2010 WHO recommendations. The ARVs currently used are in line with these guidelines. The standard ART regimens recommended in these guidelines are mostly d4T and AZT based. The WHO 2013 consolidated guidelines recommend newer regimens, which instead of d4T or AZT have TDF as the backbone.[35] NCHADS is aware of these recommendations and has started preparing for the phasing-out of d4T. TDF-based regimens are planned to be introduced for first-line treatment of adult patients in late 2013. A draft switch protocol has been developed and is expected to be disseminated around July 2013, before the arrival of TDF stocks. The programme has informed the review team that it is aware of the importance of proper planning to minimize pharmaceutical wastage through expiry or obsolescence. It is also understood that the switch of new and existing patients from d4T- to TDF-based regimens needs to be properly timed to ensure uninterrupted availability of both drugs for patients at sites and avoid any stock-outs of drugs. The team was furthermore informed that the NCHADS Forecasting Working Group conducted several analyses to better understand the clinical, cost, logistical and programmatic implications of different approaches to the switch.

Over the past years, there have been several critical stock situations, mostly as a result of delayed approval by the Global Fund of NCHADS national forecasting calculations. In our view, this can largely be improved by NCHADS adopting a more structured and well-documented forecasting approach, in which assumptions are clearly described, particularly the efforts made to validate site-level logistic data. This applies to all commodities including ARVs but, in particular, to HIV diagnostics and reagents.

The national sequential rapid testing algorithm is based on Determine HIV-1/2 assay, HIV-1/2 STAT-PAK dipstick assay, and the Uni-Gold test. The HIV tests procured by NCHADS are based on this rational and commonly used algorithm. The diagnostics and reagents procured by NCHADS for CD4 and viral load monitoring are dictated by the machines in use in the country.

The medicines supplied for OIs and STIs are not fully aligned with the MOH/NCHADS *National guidelines for the prevention and treatment of opportunistic infections among HIV-exposed and HIV-infected adults and adolescents*[15]. Some of the recommended medicines are not supplied by NCHADS. Condoms are supplied by NCHADS (with Global Fund funds), but larger quantities are procured and distributed by Central Medical Stores (CMS) from other partners such as Population Services International and the United Nations Population Fund (UNFPA). Blood safety products include blood bags, blood screening tests, gloves, etc., which are used by the blood banks in Phnom Penh and in the provinces.

National forecasting and quantification systems

The Forecasting Working Group consists of representatives from NCHADS, CHAI, WHO and UNICEF. This group is responsible for issues related to procurement and supply management of HIV programme commodities. Routine forecasting and quantification is done by the Logistics Management Unit at NCHADS, and submitted for review, feedback and endorsement by the working group. This unit has been weakened by the departure of three staff members in 2012. The unit currently consists of three NCHADS officers.

Forecasting and quantification are needed for two reasons:
- determine the quarterly replenishment deliveries at the ART sites, and
- establish what needs to be procured nationally.

The review team observed that calculations concerning ARVs are done by one of the members of the NCHADS Logistics Management Unit in collaboration with the CHAI expert(s). CHAI has been providing technical assistance through drug access focal points since 2005. In collaboration with NCHADS, an elegant (simple but effective) reporting system has been developed, in which the 61 ART sites submit quarterly Excel (spreadsheet) reports to NCHADS, showing in detail the number of adult and paediatric patients they have on each of the ART regimens. In the same spreadsheets, facilities report on stock received, consumed and remaining. Based on patient numbers and remaining stock, the spreadsheet calculates the quantity of ARVs to be supplied to the facility. This is the basis for the quarterly supply of ARVs by the CMS to each site. These reports are submitted as hard copy to the Logistic Management Unit quarterly.

The NCHADS Logistics Management Unit transcribes data from the 61 site reports (hard copies) into another spreadsheet, which shows the number of patients per ART regimen in the country. At the time of the team's visit, the report was updated until Quarter 4 of 2012, with quarter 1 of 2013 about to be completed. Table 10 shows the four most commonly used regimens (covering 87% of all adult regimens).

The Logistics Management Unit receives monthly reports of ARV drug stocks at the CMS. During the review team visit to the CMS, it was confirmed that the latest report (22 April 2013) tallied perfectly with the actual stock held at the CMS.

The Logistics Management Unit uses Excel for national forecasting. The basic approach followed for each ARV is as follows:
- Need for the coming year, based on number of patients per regimen (e.g. 1200 packs)
- PLUS 50% buffer (600 packs)
- PLUS: quantity that will be consumed in the months until the order arrives (e.g. 700)
- MINUS: Current stock in entire country (e.g. 1000), and
- MINUS: stock in pipeline (e.g. 200).

In the above example, the quantity to be procured would be: 1200 + 600 + 700 – 1000 – 200 = 1300 packages.

This is an adequate approach. The 50% buffer is added every year but since the remaining stock is subtracted, there is no risk of accumulation of buffer drugs.

Table 10: Most commonly used ART regimens, Cambodia, 2013

No.	Regimens	Number and proportion of patients treated, 2012							
		Q1		Q12		Q3		Q4	
		Number	%	Number	%	Number	%	Number	%
1	d4T (30)+3TC+NVP	16 322	37.91	16 481	37.70	16 335	36.69	16 692	36.36
2	AZT+3TC+NVP	11 601	26.94	11 868	27.15	12 323	27.68	12 736	27.74
3	d4T (30)+3TC+EFV	5 455	12.67	5 385	12.32	5 486	12.32	579	12.15
4	AZT+3TC+EFV	4 541	10.55	4 655	10.65	4 860	10.91	5 058	11.02

The review team was informed that the national ART reports did not fully tally with the quantity of ARVs consumed. This led to concern by some partners that the drugs were leaking from the system and that the reported consumption of ARVs exceeded what could be expected based on patient treatment numbers. In response to this, the team looked at the quantification of cost driving ARVs, for example: stavudine + lamivudine + nevirapine (d4T+3TC+NVP).

The NCHADS overview of all patients per regimen shows that in Quarter 4 of 2012, there were 16 692 patients using this formulation. Rounding this to 17 000 patients, we can expect that the annual need for this drug is: 17 000 patients x 365 days x 2 tablets per day = 12.4 million tablets, which is 207 000 packages of 60 tablets. Adding 50% buffer, that means 310 000 packages would be needed as a starting point for the quantification. The latest forecast presented to the Global Fund (27 September 2001) indeed assumed 309 673 packages, which tallies well with the team's expectation. The same logic could be followed in subsequent columns (subtracting the remaining stock in the country and adding quantities that would be consumed during the lead time).

The review team also checked the overall expenditure on ARVs. Assuming an average cost of ART per person per year of US$ 100 (the cheapest and most common regimens are now around US$ 65 per patient/year but US$ 100 is a fair average to make up for the more expensive second-line and paediatric regimens), and noting that the programme now has nearly 55 000 patients on ART, the value of drugs consumed per year should be around US$ 5.5 million. The latest Global Fund procurement supply management plan shows annual ARV drug values of US$ 4.6 million in 2011, US$ 5.5 million in 2012 and US$ 7.9 million in 2013. Although 2013 appears to be on the higher side (partly due to the increased use of more expensive formulations), years 2011 and 2012 were well in line with the expected overall value.

Based on these two assessments, the review team had no reason to suspect significant over-quantification or leakage of ARVs from the programme. For a possible explanation of the reported mismatch between consumption and treatment figures, see the section on "Expiry" below. Box 13 is a summary of factors concerned with ARV quantification in Cambodia.

> **Box 14: Factors affecting the quantification of ARVs in Cambodia, 2013**
>
> **What makes ARV quantification easy in Cambodia**
>
> (1) There is only one source of finance: Global Fund.
> (2) The majority of ARVs are stored at the CMS, which provides accurate stock overview reports.
> (3) ARVs are used at only 61 ART sites.
> (4) Treatment numbers are now fairly constant (no more rapid treatment expansion).
> (5) All 61 sites report quarterly on patients per regimen and remaining stock.
> (6) The majority of adult patients (around 93%) receive the standard first-line regimen.
> (7) Only 5% of adults receive the second-line regimen.
>
> **What makes ARV quantification difficult in Cambodia**
>
> (1) There is only one source of finance: Global Fund.
> (2) If anything gets delayed, there is no alternative source as back-up.

HIV diagnostics/laboratory supplies are notoriously difficult to forecast. New products are regularly introduced, there are few manufacturers, lead times are long, costs are high and shelf-lives are short. Furthermore, there are no regular detailed reports regarding usage rates at the facilities. Usage of CD4 and viral load reagents is expected to increase sharply in the coming months/years.

While the NCHADS Forecasting Working Group and Logistic Management Unit are responsible for forecasting and quantifying the HIV diagnostics and laboratory supplies, methodologies and data collection are underdeveloped.[w] The review team could not clarify when and how these commodities are forecasted or how available stocks are monitored. Nearly every facility visited by the review team during the upcountry visits reported stock-outs of HIV diagnostics such as Determine HIV-1/2 tests.

In summary, as shown in Box 14, several challenging factors complicate quantification and procurement of HIV diagnostics in Cambodia.

Medicines for treating OIs and STIs are rather difficult to forecast as there is no solid history that could be used to reliably calculate average consumption rates. Furthermore, the products needed for these treatments are also supplied from other sources such as the national budget. Meanwhile, NCHADS has committed to the Global Fund to procure these medicines through the voluntary pooled procurement mechanism. Its lead times are long and many manufacturers have minimum order quantities. Long-term forecasts are required and NCHADS needs to clearly lay out its approach to this issue.

---

[w] The NCHADS website (www.nchads.org) gives the terms of reference for various NCHADS departments, including those of the technical bureaus. Some of these are related to forecasting and quantification. Among the terms of reference for the Logistics Management Unit are the following: "To develop a national quantification system for all required items related to HIV/AIDS care and treatment (antiretroviral [ARV] and opportunistic infection [OI] medications, CD4 and VCT reagents, consumables, equipment) and the care and treatment of sexually transmitted infections (STI - medications, reagents, consumables and equipment)" and "To establish quantifications for all required items related to HIV/AIDS and STI care and treatment". However, the terms of reference for the Technical Bureau of VCT include: "To identify the needs, and ensure availability of equipment, reagents and consumables for VCT services".

> **Box 15: What makes quantification/procurement of HIV diagnostics difficult in Cambodia**
>
> (1) There is only one source of finance: the Global Fund.
> (2) Any delay or problem ▸ PROBLEM and no alternative.
> (3) There is no documented methodology showing how, when and, by whom forecasting is done, what are the assumed lead times, safety stock level, etc. This causes delays as it raises questions and concerns at the Local Fund Agent and Global Fund.
> (4) There has been scaling up of HIV testing, and CD4 and viral load monitoring.
> (5) Many products are new and unfamiliar, which leads to mistakes.
> (6) Products have a short shelf-life and high value.
> (7) The order lead time is long, especially via voluntary pooled procurement mechanisms.

Procurement mechanisms

ARVs, OI/STI medicines, condoms and HIV diagnostics/laboratory supplies that are financed by the Global Fund are procured via voluntary pooled procurement. This mechanism ensures that products are obtained from pre-qualified manufacturers at competitive prices and that procurement complies with Global Fund policies.

However, the NCHADS' procurement officer indicated several issues with voluntary pooled procurement, including long lead times and delays, complex decision-making, lengthy e-mail cascades and lack of a focal communication person. Other shortcomings were given but, in our opinion, most of these could not be attributed to this mechanism. Delayed approval by the Global Fund of procurement plans, for example, may add to the lead time but this would delay the experienced even if other procurement methods were used.

In the team's view and from experience in other countries, the voluntary pooled procurement mechanism is suitable for ARVs, condoms and major commonly used HIV diagnostics such as Determine HIV-1/2 test kits. It is generally not well suited for procurement of OI/STI medicines as these are often needed in small quantities. It would make more sense if these products were procured by the Principal Recipient from one of the international stock-keeping wholesalers such as IDA Foundation or Missionpharma.[x]

As for the larger group of HIV diagnostics and laboratory reagents (around US$ 3–4 million per year), this consists of a few big items and many small ones. Challenges include complex product specifications, short shelf-life of some items, and steep scaling up expected in CD4 and viral load testing. This makes forecasting important but difficult. It would probably work better to order such products via UNICEF as they have a local presence that can confirm specifications with NCHADS, and an office in Copenhagen with adequate procurement capacity.

Orders by the facilities

For general essential medicines, Cambodia has for many years been using a paper-based, quarterly ordering system. Around 10 years ago, a computerized stock control system was introduced at the national level and at the operational district level. The software was developed by the USAID-funded Reproductive Health and Child Alliance (RACHA).

---

[x] IDA Foundation and Missionpharma are not-for-profit suppliers of essential, quality-assured medicines and medical supplies to low- and medium-income countries.

Initially, there was no electronic data exchange between these systems. The database at the operational district level was basically used to provide the quantities to be entered on paper order forms, which were then processed through numerous steps before the CMS could act upon them.

In recent years, RACHA has introduced two additional levels to this system. The system now has four levels:
(1) NATDID (National Drug Information Database), used by the CMS;
(2) PRODID (Provincial Drug Information Database), used by the provinces;
(3) ODDID (Operational District Drug Information Database), used by the districts; and
(4) HOSDID (Hospital Drug Information Database), used by the hospitals.

The RACHA system calculates the quantities needed by a facility on the basis of average monthly consumption over the past 12 months. In the past, no correction was made for months of stock-out and this resulted in inappropriate estimation of facility needs. This has now been fixed as the system compensates for periods of stock-out when calculating the average monthly consumption. The team considers the RACHA system to be well designed and observed that RACHA provided excellent technical support to users across the country.

The traditional paper-based and RACHA ordering systems calculate needed quantities on the basis of average monthly consumption, which was not ideal for ARVs in the Cambodia situation during the scale-up phase. Therefore, NCHADS developed an Excel spreadsheet through which the ART pharmacies of the 61 ART-providing hospitals can order ARVs on a quarterly basis. This Excel sheet requires the site to enter the number of adult and paediatric patients they have on each of the ART regimens. The site also reports on the ARVs received, consumed and remaining. Excel will then calculate the quantities required for the next quarter. OI/STI drugs, condoms, condoms and HIV diagnostics/laboratory supplies needed by the hospital pharmacies are requested by the sites using separate NCHADS requisition forms, which are submitted to NCHADS as hard copies. Based on these Excel reports, NCHADS makes a quarterly distribution schedule. Once this schedule is approved by the MOH, it can be used by the CMS for the next round of distribution. It would be useful for all subpharmacies providing treatment for OIs and ART to be integrated with the HOSDID system while taking into consideration the need for both consumption and morbidity data when conducting national forecasts of ARVs and other commodities for HIV. This will free capacity in the Local Management Unit team, which could then be dedicated to other activities such as improved annual forecasting of HIV diagnostics and laboratory supplies.

Storage and distribution at the CMS

The CMS warehouse provides an adequate environment and storage conditions. It uses the NATDID inventory control system developed by RACHA. This system is working well. The CMS tracks items according to expiry date and batch number. The team confirmed that the stock levels in the NATDID system matched with the paper bin[y] cards as well as with actual physical stock. The CMS distributes products according to a fixed quarterly distribution plan. Products are issued according to FEFO (first expiry first out). From what the team observed, it concluded that the CMS may at times reduce requested quantities in response to low stock levels; but this is not a regularly occurring practice. The reported supply of additional quantities is addressed in the next section.

Expiry

Some expiry (e.g. 1–3% of annual value) occurs at even the best-run national programmes. At the time of the team's visit to the CMS, there were no Global Fund-funded ARVs or OI/STI drugs that appeared at risk of expiry (most had at least one year of remaining shelf-life). According to the CMS director, there has been no expiry at all over the past few years. The lack of any expired or obsolete products at the CMS is remarkable. We are aware that products at risk of expiry at the central level (e.g. stock with less than 6 months remaining

---

[y] Bin card is also called stock card. *See* WHO essential medicines and health products information portal at http://apps.who.int/medicinedocs/en/d/Js7919e/10.2.html#Js7919e.10.2

shelf-life) are pushed into the system and expiry is likely to occur at the health facility. Although health facilities do complain about occasionally receiving products with near-expiry dates, sometimes in excess of what they ordered, we believe this has not occurred at a significant scale with ARVs. Assuming that a 2% loss due to expiry/obsolescence would be acceptable, in the case of Cambodia's ARVs, this would mean 2% of 55 000 patient treatments, or around 1100 patients. At an average annual treatment cost of US$ 100, this would mean a value of around US$ 110 000 or a total of US$ 5.5 million for ARVs. The review team considers this acceptable and this calculation would help refute the alleged mismatch between reported consumption and numbers of patients/treatment/year signalled to us by some partners.

Stock-out mitigation

In case a critical stock situation occurs at a facility, they can contact NCHADS. NCHADS may then arrange an urgent delivery/collection from the emergency stock kept at NCHADS or CMS, or contact a neighbouring site and request that they share some of their stock.

However, when a critical stock situation occurs at the national level, the options are fairly limited. In other countries, there may be parallel programmes such as the US President's Emergency Plan for AIDS Relief (PEPFAR), national budget, and other programmes that can be asked to help out but in Cambodia, all ARVs are financed by the Global Fund and are procured via voluntary pooled procurement, which has long lead times. In some cases, the only option for avoiding treatment interruption will be to switch some patients to another regimen.

Recommendations

8.1 NCHADS' approach to national forecasting for ARVs is sound; but the methodology used, including responsibilities, data flow, assumptions and timings, needs to be better documented and informed by evidence and experience. Doing so would help reduce the Global Fund's anxiety over possible misquantification and, therefore, speed up order approvals. The method would need to take into account the longer lead times of the voluntary pooled procurement mechanism and set appropriate safety stock levels.

8.2 NCHADS may consider engaging a laboratory specialist to develop a documented method for, and lead the forecasting and monitoring of, HIV diagnostics/laboratory supplies.

8.3 NCHADS may continue using voluntary pooled procurement to procure pre-qualified ARVs and other large-value items at competitive prices in compliance with the Global Fund procurement rules. However, alternative mechanisms acceptable to the Global Fund need to be identified to procure the wide range of OI/STI medicines, HIV diagnostics and laboratory consumables required by the programme in smaller quantities. Options could be an agreement with an international wholesaler or with UNICEF.

8.4 It is suggested that NCHADS and USAID-funded RACHA collaborate towards integrating NCHADS Excel-based ordering system into the HOSDID system used for essential drugs. This may require a switch from the current patient-based order system to an average consumption approach. While the RACHA system may require some site-specific adjustments, especially for less commonly used products such as second-line ARVs, the system is robust enough to handle the majority of needed supplies. Doing so would reduce the workload at the NCHADS Local Management Unit, which can then focus on more strategic national forecasting challenges.

9. Blood safety

The National Blood Transfusion Center, within the MOH is, the highest authority responsible for the organization and supervision of blood safety in the country. The National Blood Transfusion Center oversees 21 provincial blood banks and blood services within the private sector. Regional blood services at the provincial hospitals of Battambang, Kampong Cham and Siem Reap are in the process of being established or planned. In 2011-2012, PEPFAR funded a one-year technical assistance programme in collaboration with the MOH, National Blood Transfusion Center and US CDC to assess the current situation of the Cambodian blood system.[6] The comprehensive assessment covered national and provincial governance, policy and legislation; blood service operations at the National Blood Transfusion Center and 21 provincial blood transfusion centres; and clinical interfaces with hospitals (public, private and not-for-profit). Recommendations were included in the design of the National Strategic Plan for National Transfusion Services (2013–2017), which provides a road map for action to consolidate and strengthen the quality of blood transfusion services in the nation.[75] Current funding sources for blood safety activities comprise the MOH (80%) and Global Fund (20%), with ad-hoc funding by the US CDC and WHO for specific activities.

Laboratory screening of blood donations for transfusion-transmitted infections (TTIs) is routinely done (Table 11). However, there are sporadic reports of stock-outs of test kits. While the proportion of voluntary non-remunerated blood donors has improved in the past year, it remains unacceptably low. In 2012, 48 298 blood units were screened for TTIs; 34 508 (71.4%) were family replacement donors and 13 790 (28.6%) voluntary non-remunerated donors from static and mobile blood banks.

In the National Blood Transfusion Center, enzyme-linked immunosorbent assay (ELISA) is used for HIV screening while in the provincial blood banks, an HIV rapid test is used. Similarly, screening for hepatitis B and hepatitis C viruses is done by using rapid tests, while syphilis screening is performed using a RPR test RPR and confirmed by a TPHA test. Quality assurance for the tests is conducted by the National Institute of Public Health reference laboratory, with future plans to include external quality assurance from WHO regional laboratories. There have been discussions with NCHADS to re-allocate their ELISA machines (previously for HIV testing) to blood banks.

Table 11: Results of testing of blood units for TTIs, National Blood Transfusion Center, 2012

Screening test	Prevalence in % (total N = 48 298)
HIV	0.35
Hepatitis B virus	6.2
Hepatitis C virus	0.87
Syphilis	0.89
Malaria	0.012

Recommendations

9.1 The review team endorses the recommendations made by the 2012 comprehensive assessment of blood transfusion services, and supports their early implementation.

9.2 The National Blood Transfusion Center may consider strengthening procurement and supply management of test kits for TTIs (HIV, Hepatitis B virus, Hepatitis C virus, syphilis), in line with recommendation 8.2.

9.3 The National Blood Transfusion Centre, NCHADS and the National Reference Laboratory are advised to strengthen coordination to ensure EQAS for test kits in the programme, in line with recommendation 7.3.

10. Sustainable financing for the HIV/AIDS response

Cambodia has shown steady economic growth over the past decade, and experienced growth rates of 6–13% except in 2009. In 2012, its gross domestic product (GDP) per capita was estimated at US$ 926 in current US$ and 2395 in current international dollars based on purchasing power parity (PPP).[76] Of the social sector, health and education were projected to have the largest increases in budget spending with their estimated annual growth comparable to that of other industries, such as manufacturing, trade and services.[77]

Total expenditure on health in Cambodia increased from US$ 564 million in 2008 to US$ 763 million in 2012 (Table 12). During the same period, general government health expenditure increased from US$ 105 million to US$ 187 million. In 2012, general government health expenditure accounted for 1.3% of GDP. Of the total health expenditure, general government health expenditure accounted for 24.6%, while external expenditure and out-of-pocket health expenditure constituted 15.3% and 61.5%, respectively.

Table 12: Health expenditure in Cambodia, 2008–2012

Health financing indicators	2008	2009	2010	2011	2012
Total health expenditure (US$ millions)	564	651	678	712	763
Total health expenditure per capita (US$)	41	46	47	49	52
General government health expenditure (US$ millions)	105	125	152	162	187
General government health expenditure per capita (US$)	8	9	11	12	13
Total health expenditure as % of GDP	5.5	6.3	5.8	5.5	5.4
General government health expenditure as % of GDP	1.1	1.1	1.3	1.3	1.3
General government health expenditure as % of total health expenditure	19.0	19.8	22.8	23.6	24.6
External expenditure on health (US$ millions)	111	128	108	107	117
External expenditure on health per capita (US$)	8	9	8	7	8
External expenditure on health as % of total health expenditure	19.7	19.7	15.9	15.0	15.3
Out-of-pocket expenditure on health (US$ millions)	347	394	416	444	469
Out-of-pocket expenditure on health per capita (US$)	25	28	29	31.0	32
Out-of-pocket expenditure on health as % of total health expenditure	61.5	60.5	61.4	62.4	61.5

Source: Kingdom of Cambodia, Ministry of Health, 2013
Note: Estimates in US$ millions are rounded to the nearest million.

In 2012, 87% of Cambodia's HIV/AIDS programme was funded by external sources – United Nations, Global Fund, bilateral and international nongovernment organizations,[78] and other multilateral organizations. Reliance on external funding and the unpredictability of continued funding beyond 2015 pose urgent threats to the sustainability of the HIV/AIDS programme in Cambodia.

As shown in Table 13, total HIV/AIDS expenditure declined from US$ 58.1 million in 2010 to US$ 50.9 million in 2012. Government expenditure on HIV/AIDS was 11% of the total HIV/AIDS expenditure at US$ 5.7 million in 2012 (Figure 17).

Table 13: Expenditure on HIV/AIDS in Cambodia, 2008–2012

HIV/AIDS financing indicators	2008	2009	2010	2011	2012
Total HIV/AIDS expenditure (US$ millions)	51.8	53.7	58.1	53.2	50.9
Government HIV/AIDS expenditure (US$ millions)	5.3	1.7	2.4	5.6*	5.7
External HIV/AIDS expenditure (US$ millions)	46.6	52.0	55.6	46.6	44.3
Total HIV/AIDS expenditure as % of total health expenditure	9.2	8.2	8.6	7.5	6.7
Government HIV/AIDS expenditure as % of total HIV/AIDS expenditure	10.2	3.2	4.1	10.5	11.2
Government HIV/AIDS expenditure as % of general government health expenditure	5.0	1.4	1.6	3.5	3.0
External HIV/AIDS expenditure as % of total HIV/AIDS expenditure	90.0	96.8	95.7	87.6	87.0
External HIV/AIDS expenditure as % of total external health expenditure	42.0	40.6	51.5	43.6	37.9

Source: National AIDS Spending Assessments II, III and IV; Kingdom of Cambodia, Ministry of Health, 2013
Note: Estimates in US$ millions are rounded to the nearest tenth of a million.
*Government HIV/AIDS expenditure for 2011 and 2012 include information on government salaries, which were not obtained for previous years.

About US$ 2.5 million in government salaries for health workers working full-time on HIV/AIDS were not accounted for in the National AIDS Spending Assessment III for 2009 and 2010.[78] Considering this exclusion in 2009 and 2010, government expenditure on HIV/AIDS has remained fairly constant since 2007 in absolute terms. Only 3% of general government expenditure on health is for HIV/AIDS, while 38% of total external funding for health is allocated to HIV/AIDS. It should be noted that while only 60% of the total 106 organizations requested to submit expenditure information responded with HIV/AIDS expenditure data,[78] the data available are estimated to represent the majority of total spending.

Given the unpredictability of external funding beyond the current fiscal year, there is an urgent need to prepare a resource mobilization plan for sustained funding of essential HIV/AIDS services until 2020. This should take into consideration the current low government expenditure on health and priority of other programmes. As Cambodia's economy continues to grow, it will soon become a lower–middle-income country and face increased counterpart financing requirements by the Global Fund from the change in income status. Of the total expenditure on HIV/AIDS, government expenditure is 11.2%. For the current grant renewal process, the Global Fund requires low-income countries to satisfy a 5% minimum threshold where government contribution to the programme is at least 5% of the sum of government and Global Fund contributions to the programme. This counterpart financing threshold also applies to the new funding model. For 2012, Cambodia's government contribution is 22.2% of the sum of government and Global Fund contributions to the programme, thus satisfying the minimum threshold.

Findings and Recommendations

Figure 17: HIV/AIDS spending by financing sources, 2009–2012

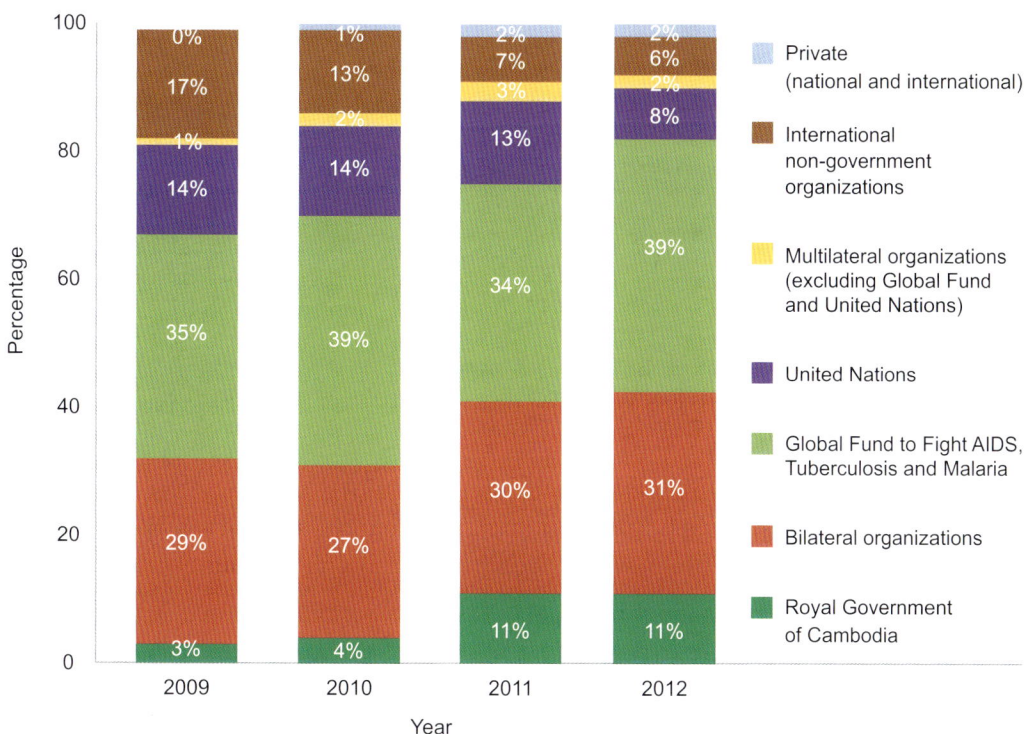

Source: National AIDS Spending Assessments II, III and IV; Kingdom of Cambodia, Ministry of Health, 2013

In Cambodia's efforts to eliminate the transmission of HIV infection by 2020, it is critical for the country to improve coordination between donors, development partners and the government to sustain funding for essential HIV/AIDS services, in line with its current Health Strategic Plan 2008–2015, Strategic Framework for Health Financing 2008–2015, and future plans. Donors have the responsibility to avoid sudden withdrawal of funding and support the HIV/AIDS programme at adequate levels while more diverse funding mechanisms are sought. During this period, the government will need to gradually increase its expenditure on health through various financing mechanisms as part of the long-term integration of the HIV/AIDS programme in the broader health system. Transparency and accountability as well as commitment by all stakeholders – government, donors and development partners – are essential for ensuring that the HIV/AIDS programme is financially sustainable and able to maintain the continuum of key prevention, care and treatment programmes. The elimination of new HIV infections may also reduce costs in the long run.

New knowledge is needed to inform strategic priority-settings. Current ongoing or completed studies include the following: National AIDS Spending Assessment IV, budgeting for the Global Fund HIV single stream funding grant phase 2 and costing for Cambodia 3.0. Evidence that needs to be further developed involves effectiveness and efficiency assessments, unit costs and resource needs estimates. In particular, unit costs for some HIV/AIDS services, such as the actual cost per sex worker reached or cost per STI treatment, have been established and improved; however, these unit costs are costs per output and not per outcome.[79,80] Through the generation and use of evidence on the costs of HIV prevention, the targeting of key populations most at risk may also be improved.

Mechanisms to increase domestic funding through supply-side financing (e.g. ARVs, condoms, HIV testing) and demand-side financing (e.g. inclusion of ART, STI services in social health protection schemes) are emerging developments in Cambodia's health financing policy to move towards universal health coverage. Demand-side financing of social health protection schemes, such as Health Equity Funds and National Social Security Funds, may complement current supply-side financing. Health Equity Funds are expected to be implemented nationally by 2015. Costs of implementation are currently being estimated. As of now, 60% of Health Equity Funds are donor financed and 40% government financed. Fragmentation and reliance on donor funding of financing schemes continue to remain as challenges to the country's overall financing strategy to increase population coverage, especially for poor and vulnerable populations.

The programme can use its multi-year plan to advocate and work with development partners, the MOH, Ministry of Economy and Finance, other ministries and other entities. With the Global Fund's new funding model, countries are required to decide on their programme allocations for HIV/AIDS, TB, malaria, and possibly health systems strengthening from a shared envelope. The role of the Country Coordinating Committee will be critical to ensuring that there is coordination and consensus among donors, development partners and the government on what the priorities are for each programme and health systems strengthening and how best to allocate funds across the different activities.

The systematic monitoring and evaluation by NCHADS of its own budget, and the effectiveness and efficiency of each aspect of the programme over time should enable the programme to better determine how to increase value for money by improving efficiencies in each area. The annual review for the Global Fund grant can be used as an opportunity to review all activities, regardless of funder, and to assess activities in further detail beyond the purpose of the Global Fund review. As an example of the benefits of routine monitoring and evaluation, procurement delays and forecasting issues discussed in Section 9 may also be addressed by shifting funds that have not been used to procure medicines and supplies in advance of the current schedule. In addition, continued progress can be made towards expanding links to the health system based on the review's recommendations to improve the efficiencies of specific aspects of the programme.

Recommendations

10.1 For informing priority-setting and maximizing value for money to serve as key inputs to the multi-year strategic plan, it would be necessary to generate and use evidence. The strategic plan would have to include a resource needs and mobilization plan. The programme could increase value for money by allocating resources to the most effective programmes and improving service delivery and management efficiencies in informing the prioritization of essential HIV/AIDS services for its resource needs and mobilization plan, given its absorptive capacity.

10.2 It is important to routinely monitor and evaluate the funding and expenditure levels, resource allocations and efficiency of the programme, including how to gradually increase linkages with other entities in the health system.

10.3 Domestic funding can be increased through supply- (e.g. ARVs, condoms, HIV testing) and demand-side financing (e.g. inclusion of ART, STI services in social health protection schemes). It is important to assess mechanisms to achieve this as part of emerging developments in Cambodia's health financing policy to move towards universal health coverage.

10.4 NCHADS should be actively involved and engaged in the development of the Cambodia health strategic plan and health financing policy, which are in the early stages of development. These measures will constitute a major step towards long-term sustainability and expanded linkages of the HIV programme to the health system.

General conclusions and summary

Upon careful and systematic examination of past achievements, current capacities, status and trends, the review team focused its attention on the two key questions that it was asked to address:

(1) Is the national response to HIV progressing satisfactorily towards its 2015 objectives?
(2) Is the country on track for eliminating new HIV infections by 2020?

In order to underpin its conclusions, the review team considered the following rationale:

1. Cambodia has a solid record of a dynamic and effective response to HIV and the potential to progress further:

- Cambodia has received credit for having curbed the HIV epidemic, which began to spread in the country in the 1990s, and for having rapidly introduced and scaled up prevention programmes among sex workers, programmes to prevent mother-to-child transmission of HIV and access to ART for people living with HIV.

- Cambodia is one of the few countries to have successfully reversed its HIV epidemic, as reflected by an estimated HIV prevalence that fell from 1.7% in adults aged 15–49 years in 1998 to 0.76% in 2012. The estimated number of new HIV infections has reduced from 20 000 per year in the mid-1990s to around 2100 by 2009 and 1400 by 2012.

- In 2012, NCHADS estimated that over 72 000 people aged 15 years and older were living with HIV in Cambodia, 39 000 of whom (54%) were women, pointing to a gender differential in the likelihood of acquiring HIV infection in the country. NCHADS estimated that 53 000 individuals older than 15 years, including 28 000 women, were eligible for ART (as defined by a CD4 count of <350 cells/μL). By 30 June 2012, the national programme was providing ART to 43 285 (81%) adults living with HIV and reported low loss to follow-up or death at 12 months (7%), 24 months (16%) and 5 years (22%), while 7081 people living with HIV were actively followed in pre-ART care. The nationwide facility ART report indicates that by the end of the 2012, 48 913 adults and children were receiving ART.

- The reduction in new HIV infections and prevalence is mirrored by the decreasing HIV prevalence among newly registered TB cases. Routine programme data show that HIV prevalence among TB patients declined from 13% in 2009 to 4.4% in 2012, a threefold decrease. HIV testing rates among newly registered TB patients increased from 70% in 2009 to 80% in 2012. The proportion of TB/HIV coinfected individuals starting on ART increased from 14% in 2009 to 89% in 2012. TB screening coverage among people living with HIV was 85% in 2012, short of the 95% target set for that year. Of the 3411 people living with HIV screened for TB, 27% had active TB. The TB epidemic is now evolving independently from the HIV epidemic. However, TB is still a significant cause of co-morbidity among people living with HIV.

- Today, rather than becoming complacent about the successes achieved in the past and the benefits they have yielded for the whole population, Cambodia is contemplating a higher challenge: it has committed itself to the elimination of transmission of HIV in the country by 2020. The country has set for itself ambitious targets: (i) to reduce estimated HIV incidence among the population aged 15 years and older from 18/100 000 in 2010 to 3/100 000 or less by 2020; (ii) to reduce the HIV transmission rate from HIV-positive mothers to their infants from 13% in 2010 to 2% or less by 2020; and (iii) to increase syphilis screening and treatment to over 95% among pregnant women by 2020.

> Having reviewed the available data, documents and reports, and carried out on-site observations and interviews, the Review of the National Health Sector Response to HIV concluded that Cambodia was on track to achieve its 2015 objectives and its ambitious goal of eliminating new HIV infections in the country by 2020. Given the level of national commitment to, and the past and current performances of, the health sector's response to HIV in Cambodia, potential obstacles to eliminate HIV transmission by 2020 are surmountable.

2. To surmount these obstacles, the following conditions will have to be met in order to achieve the 2020 HIV transmission elimination goal:

- **Sustained structures, capacities and services dedicated to HIV and STI prevention, care and treatment, and the early diagnosis and treatment of HIV/TB coinfection**
  NCHADS has served as the backbone of the national response to HIV since its establishment in 1998. The remarkable strength of the structure lies in the combined product of strong leadership, use of evidence in strategic vision, availability of a panoply of standard operating procedures disseminated across the health system, a well-trained and skilled staff, a streamlined chain of communication with the periphery, an efficient monitoring system, and an adequate flow of financial resources. Boosting all of these assets will make HIV elimination possible.

- **Better access to services by the most vulnerable and key-affected populations (including entertainment workers, female and male sex workers, men who have sex with men, transsexual and transgender persons, and drug users) in a supportive legal and policy environment**
  The current policy and legal environment is partly conducive to open access to services by key-affected populations. The 2002 HIV law is sound from a public health perspective. Unfortunately, the 2007 law on combating sex trafficking and the 2010 policy on safer communities, while well intended, have exacerbated the vulnerability of those sex workers and drug users who refrain from accessing HIV services due to fear of harassment or arrest. The interpretation and application of the 2007 law and the 2010 policy by commune leaders, law enforcement agents and lawyers need to be aligned with the goal of improving public security and public health, as one cannot be realized if the other is not. The effects of the law and policy need to be evaluated from a dual HIV and public security perspective. Future laws and policies aimed at reinforcing public security should be subjected to a health impact assessment, carried out, before their enactment, jointly by the MOH and the Ministry of Interior. Of equal importance, further support of the Police–Community Partnership Initiative will need to be effectively scaled up and closely monitored from the triple perspective of: (i) its effectiveness as a means of reducing the risk and impact of HIV; (ii) its compliance with public health best practice, ethical principles and human rights norms and standards; and (iii) its adherence to the terms of the 2002 Cambodian HIV law.

  Discrimination against people living with HIV or people assumed to be at higher-than-average risk of acquiring infection (key-affected populations) is reported to have declined in the past two decades but has not been eliminated, in particular, for women attending reproductive health services. The training and retraining of health personnel on best health practices in the context of HIV, with particular reference to the 2002 Cambodian HIV law, is a requisite for eliminating HIV-related discrimination, which is itself a requisite for eliminating HIV transmission by 2020.

- **Stronger follow-up along the cascade of services, from creation of and demand for voluntary HIV testing and counselling to sustained and efficiently monitored use of care and treatment, devoting particular attention to gender issues, age and key-affected populations**
Losses along the CoC cascade do occur, and this reduces the impact of the programme. High mortality rates and loss to follow up occur among pre-ART patients who have not yet been initiated on treatment. Current systems to link HIV-infected individuals from HIV testing to care and treatment and track them are suboptimal. These gaps need be corrected before and beyond 2020 to increase the efficiency of services and ultimately to monitor and evaluate the dual benefit of ART programmes, both reduction of mortality and new infections. The infrastructures and services for HIV testing and treatment are in place. With a few adjustments, the programme can focus on identifying the few new HIV infections and start earlier treatment through better linking of targeted prevention services to care, and expansion of partner testing of HIV-positive individuals, in particular, HIV-positive pregnant women. Measuring the cascade will be facilitated by the introduction of a unique identifier assigned to people living with HIV for the purpose of linking of their various health records and facilitating follow-up of the continuum of prevention, care and treatment. The testing and introduction of such a system should be accompanied by measures to restrict access to the electronic database, while enhancing the capacity of persons entered in the database to access complaint and redressal mechanisms in the event of intentional or inadvertent unauthorized access and breaches of confidentiality.

- **Sharper epidemiological targeting and more effective interventions at sufficient intensity and scale, identifying the few new HIV infections and introducing earlier treatment to harness the dual benefit of mortality reduction and prevention of further spread among those at highest risk**
Current interventions under the Boosted Continuum of Prevention to Care and Treatment are reaching large numbers of individuals in broadly defined risk groups, yet evidence suggests that coverage may be insufficient for marginalized and highly vulnerable subpopulations with overlapping high-risk behaviours. As a result, new HIV and sexually transmitted infections can be expected to spread at high rates among, for example, drug-injecting women, men who have sex with men and transgender persons who sell sex, "hidden" sex workers working outside entertainment establishments, and individuals with varied risks who move in and out of prison or detention centres. Suboptimal intervention coverage within most-affected communities and almost complete absence of prevention interventions in closed settings may easily account for several hundred new HIV infections per year, unless these apparent prevention gaps are filled. The identification of new pockets of high transmission and continued monitoring of the response in known high transmission networks is a prerequisite for eliminating new infections.

- **Expanded access to, and voluntary use of, HIV counselling and testing by pregnant women attending antenatal clinics with full and timely provision of ART for life during pregnancy and/or shortly before delivery to protect their offspring from HIV infection**
The country is poised to implement the elimination of mother-to-child transmission initiative based on the new option B+ strategy, which is provision of lifelong ART for all pregnant women who test HIV positive, linking prevention to care and treatment services for key-affected populations and starting treatment for prevention among serodiscordant couples (i.e. when one partner is HIV-infected and the other not). These interventions are being scaled up and, within seven years, would have been implemented nationwide. Measuring the cascade of services and following pregnant women transitioning between maternal and child health and ART services will be essential to not only improve the efficiency of services, but also to monitor and evaluate the impact of the programme. The infrastructure and systems for achieving this are in place and could, with a little adjustment, allow this effort if resources are sustained. Both the concept note on Treatment as Prevention (TasP) and the new Cambodia 3.0 Conceptual Framework were developed before the couples counselling guideline and the 2013 WHO ART guidelines were released. There is now an opportunity to align the Cambodia 3.0 strategic vision and TasP concept note with these WHO guidelines.

- **Greater synergy within the health sector and across other sectors of development**
Reinforced linkages to other programmes/initiatives within the health sector (in particular, maternal and child health, TB, mental health, primary health care, health information) will enhance the continuum of prevention, care and treatment on the basis of a clear division of roles and tasks, along with the sharing of resources needed to foster and sustain such collaboration. Similarly, governmental and civil society organizations need to strengthen their collaboration further through strategic alignment and mutual accountability. In particular, the interactions between government health centres and nongovernmental providers of community services, and links between public services and key-affected populations and people living with HIV need greater coordination and information-sharing. People living with HIV contribute to peer education and community-based care and treatment. Their expanded involvement in the formulation, implementation, and monitoring of policies and programmes concerning their health and quality of life will be a major asset in ensuring an efficient cascade of services.

    The contribution of government sectors outside health to the national response to HIV adds opportunities for achieving the elimination of HIV transmission by 2020. A review of this contribution (mid-term review of the national multisectoral strategy on HIV/AIDS) is due to take place at the end of 2013 under the auspices of the National AIDS Authority, upon which recommendations will be made to optimize responses to HIV through diverse sectors concerned with human development.

- **Greater support to health personnel through improved salary, skills upgradation and incentives to ensure staff retention and protection of the health of the Cambodian population against brain drain and the loss of those who care for them**
In the health sector, staff rotation and loss are high and likely to rise as a result of the stalling of government salaries, emergence of more competitive employment alternatives and discontinuation of staff incentives. Achieving the 2020 elimination goal requires greater stability in the deployment of human resources for health, the availability of a more attractive income scale and the creation of incentives, preferably performance based. As these issues involve changes in the civil service employment and remuneration schemes, they will not be fully resolved single-handedly by the MOH, but the Ministry may draw the attention of government leadership to the negative impacts that human resources issues may have on the response to HIV, established as a national priority.

- **Sustained external financing and a growing financial share from national sources**
In 2012, the total HIV/AIDS expenditure in the country declined from US$ 58 million in 2010 to US$ 51 million in 2012, all sources combined. Domestic public expenditure on HIV/AIDS represented 11% of this amount. In that same year, 87% of these expenditures were funded from outside sources: multilateral and bilateral official development assistance agencies, international funds and other nongovernmental organizations. Outside sources are responding to the ongoing global economic crisis by reducing the predictable volume of development aid and by encouraging countries to search for efficiencies and further adjust expenditures to evolving needs. Now is the time for the MOH and other concerned government entities (Ministry of Economy and Finance, Ministry of Planning, among others) to enhance the efficiency of the national health sector response to HIV, increase the national public share of the HIV/AIDS/STI budget, diversify external funding sources, and prepare a contingency plan for mitigating unforeseen funding shortage.

References

[1] Cambodia takes MDG prize for excellence in its AIDS response. Geneva: UNAIDS; 2010 (http://unaidstoday.org/?p=848, accessed 22 July 2013).

[2] International HIV/AIDS Alliance/KHANA. An evaluation of the MOH/NGO home care programme for people with HIV/AIDS in Cambodia. International HIV/AIDS Alliance; 2010 (http://www.hivpolicy.org/Library/HPP000305.pdf, accessed 12 November 2013).

[3] NCHADS, UNAIDS, WHO and DFID. Report of the mid-term assessment of the Ministry of Health Strategic Plan for HIV/AIDS and STDs Prevention and Care in Cambodia, 2001–2005. Phnom Penh: NCHADS. (Available on request from NCHADS)

[4] Dhaliwal M et al. Cambodia's continuum of care for people living with HIV programme: assessment of quality and cost effectiveness. London: DFID Health Resource Centre; October 2007.

[5] Cambodia joint PMTCT program review: findings and recommendations. Phnom Penh: National Maternal and Child Health Centre, Ministry of Health Cambodia; 2007.

[6] Waters N et al. Strategic improvement of Cambodia national blood transfusion services: report of the Cambodia NBTC current situation, gap analysis and recommendations. Phnomh Penh: Australian Red Cross and Blood Service; 2012.

[7] Ministry of Health, Cambodia et al. Joint review of the national TB program. Phnom Penh: World Health Organization; 2–15 August 2012.

[8] Frieson KG et al. A gender analysis of the Cambodian health sector. Phnom Penh: AusAID, Government of Cambodia, World Health Organization; 2011:6.

[9] Cambodia country brief; HIV and key affected women and girls. Bangkok: United Nations Entity for Gender Equality and the Empowerment of Women, Regional Office for Asia and the Pacific, United Nations; March 2013 (http://www.aidsdatahub.org/dmdocuments/Country_Brief_Cambodia.pdf, accessed 20 July 2013).

[10] National AIDS Authority, Cambodia. Cambodia country progress report 2012: monitoring the progress towards the implementation of the Declaration of Commitment on HIV and AIDS. Reporting period January 2010–December 2011 (http://www.unaids.org/en/dataanalysis/knowyourresponse/countryprogressreports/2012countries/ce_KH_Narrative_Report[1].pdf, accessed 20 July 2013).

[11] Chhorvann C, Vonthanak S. Estimations and projections of HIV/AIDS in Cambodia 2010–2015. Phnom Penh: NCHADS, Ministry of Health; 2011 (http://www.nchads.org/Publication/HSS/Estimations%20 and%20Projections%20of%20HIV-AIDS%20in%20Cambodia%202010-2015_eng.pdf, accessed13 November 2013).

[12] Family Health International (FHI). Behavioral surveillance surveys (BSS) guidelines for repeated behavioral surveys in populations at risk of HIV. Arlington, VA: FHI; 2000.

[13] Chhea C, Seguy N, Chan N. Integrated behavioral and biological sentinel survey: HIV prevalence among drug users in Cambodia, 2007. Phnom Penh: National Center for HIV/AIDS, Dermatology and STDs, Ministry of Health and National Authority for Combating Drugs.

[14] Sopheab H, Morineau G, Neal JJ, Chhorvann C. 2005 Cambodia STI prevalence survey: integrated biological and behavioral survey. Phnom Penh: National Center for HIV/AIDS, Dermatology and STDs, Ministry of Health.

[15] National Center for HIV/AIDS, Dermatology and STDs. National guidelines for the prevention and treatment of opportunistic infection among HIV-exposed and HIV-infected adults and adolescents, first edition. Phnom Penh: Ministry of Health, Kingdom of Cambodia; January 2012 (http://www.nchads.org/Guideline/OI%20Guideline%20for%20HIV-EI_Adults_Adol%202012%20Eng.pdf, accessed 20 July 2013).

[16] National Center for HIV/AIDS, Dermatology and STD. Annual report 2011 (http://www.nchads.org/Report/Annual%20Report%202011%20Eng.pdf, accessed12 November 2013).

[17] Sobheap H, Neal JJ, Chhorvann C. 2005 Cambodia STI prevalence survey. Sexually transmitted infections and related behaviors among brothel-based female sex workers, police, and men who have sex with men. Phnom Penh: National Center for HIV/AIDS Dermatology and STD, Ministry of Health; April 2008.

[18] National Center for HIV/AIDS, Dermatology and STDs. Conceptual framework for elimination of new HIV infections in Cambodia by 2020 as part of the health sector response towards "Three Zeros" ("Cambodia 3.0"). Phnom Penh: Ministry of Health, November 2012.

[19] National AIDS Authority. The national strategic plan for comprehensive and multisectoral response to HIV/AIDS III (2011–2015). Phnom Penh: September 2010.

[20] National Center for HIV/AIDS, Dermatology and STDs. Strategic plan for HIV/AIDS and STI prevention and care in the health sector, 2011–2015. Phnom Penh: Ministry of Health; June 2011.

[21] UNAIDS/WHO. Estimating national adult prevalence of HIV-1 in concentrated epidemics. Draft Manual EPP Version Q; May 2009:4–6 (https://www.unaids.org/en/media/unaids/contentassets/dataimport/pub/agenda/2009/20090512_epp_concepi_2009_draft_en.pdf, accessed12 November 2013).

[22] National Assembly, Cambodia. The Law on the Prevention and Control of HIV/AIDS. Phnom Penh: 26 July 2002 (http://www.ilo.org/wcmsp5/groups/public/---ed_protect/---protrav/---ilo_aids/documents/legaldocument/wcms_113128.pdf, informal English version accessed 20 July 2013).

[23] Pearshouse R. Cambodia: human trafficking legislation threatens HIV response. HIV AIDS Policy and Law Review. 2008;13(2–3):21–2.

[24] Busza J. Having the rug pulled from under your feet: one project's experience of the US policy reversal on sex work. Health Policy Plan. 2006;21(4):329–32.

[25] Union Aid Abroad – APHEDA, on behalf of the International Labour Organization (ILO), DWT for East and South-East Asia and the Pacific. Cambodia – addressing HIV vulnerabilities of indirect sex workers during the financial crisis: situation analysis, strategies and entry points for HIV/AIDS workplace education. Bangkok: ILO; 2011 (http://www.ilo.org/wcmsp5/groups/public/---asia/---ro-bangkok/documents/genericdocument/wcms_165487.pdf, accessed 20 July 2013).

[26] National Laws and Agreements Cambodia. Law on Suppression of Human Trafficking and Sexual Exploitation 2007 (http://www.no-trafficking.org/resources_laws_cambodia.html, accessed 13 December 2013).

[27] Ministry of Interior, Royal Government of Cambodia. Safety village commune/Sangkat policy guideline. Issued in Phnom Penh by the Co-Minister of the Ministry of Interior on 16 August 2010 (http://www.sithi.org/admin/upload/law/Village%20Commune%20Safety%20Policy%20(Eng)%20-%202010.pdf , English version accessed 12 November 2013).

[28] National Center for HIV/AIDS, Dermatology and STDs. HIV sentinel surveys 2010. Phnom Penh, Ministry of Health; 2012. (Available on request)

[29] National AIDS Authority. A situation and response analysis of HIV and AIDS in Cambodia. Phnom Penh: NAA; June 2010.

[30] National Authority for Combating Drugs. Report on illicit drug data and routine surveillance systems in Cambodia. Phnom Penh: United National Office for Drug and Crime; 2008 (http://www.unodc.org/documents/southeastasiaandpacific//Publications/Projects/NACD_Annual_report2007.pdf, accessed 13 December 2013).

[31] Ryan C, Ouk V, Gorbach P, Leng H, Berlioz-Arthaud A, Whittington W, et al. Explosive spread of HIV-1 and sexually transmitted disease in Cambodia. Lancet. 1998; 351:1175.

[32] Kim AA, Sun LP, Chhorvann C, Lindan C, Van Griensven F, Kilmarx PH et al. High prevalence of HIV and sexually transmitted infections among indirect sex workers in Cambodia. Sex Transm Dis. 2005:32(12):745–51.

[33] Liu K, Chhorvann C. Bros Khmer: behavioral risks on-site serosurvey among at-risk urban men in Cambodia. Phnom Penh: FHI 360/NCHADS; 2010.

[34] Lama JR et al; for the Peruvian HIV Sentinel Surveillance Working Group. Linking HIV and antiretroviral drug resistance surveillance in Peru: a model for a third-generation HIV sentinel surveillance. J Acquir Immune Defic Syndr., 2006;42(4):501–5.

[35] Consolidated guidelines on the use of antiretroviral drugs for treating and preventing HIV infection: recommendations for a public health approach. Geneva: WHO; 2013 (http://www.who.int/hiv/pub/guidelines/arv2013/download/en/index.html, accessed 13 December 2013).

[36] Guide for monitoring and evaluating national HIV testing and counselling (HTC) programmes. Geneva: WHO. Field-test version. (http://whqlibdoc.who.int/publications/2011/9789241501347_eng.pdf, accessed 13 December 2013).

[37] National Center for HIV/AIDS, Dermatology and STDs. HIV sentinel surveys 2010: female entertainment workers (FEWs) and antenatal care clinic (ANC) attendees. (Internal document. Available on request from NCHADS)

[38] WHO/UNAIDS. When and how to use assays for recent infection to estimate HIV incidence at a population level (2011). Geneva: World Health Organization; 2013 (http://www.who.int/hiv/pub/surveillance/sti_surveillance/en/index.html, accessed 13 December 2013).

[39] UNAIDS/WHO Working Group on Global HIV/AIDS and STI Surveillance. Technical Guidance Note: HIV prevalence measurement in national household surveys for countries with low HIV prevalence. December 2010 (http://www.unaids.org/en/media/unaids/contentassets/documents/epidemiology/20101207_HIVtesting_in_surveys_WG_en.pdf, accessed 12 November 2013).

[40] Guidelines on estimating the size of populations most at risk to HIV. Geneva: WHO; 2010 (http://www.who.int/hiv/pub/surveillance/estimating_populations_HIV_risk/en/, accessed 12 November 2013).

[41] National Center for HIV/AIDS, Dermatology and STDs. Conceptual framework for elimination of new HIV infections in Cambodia by 2020. Phnom Penh, Cambodia; November 2012. (Available on request)

[42] Boosted Continuum of Prevention to Care and Treatment. Phnom Penh, Cambodia: National Center for HIV/AIDS Dermatology and STD; 2013. (http://www.nchads.org/SOPs/Book%20CoPCT%20English.pdf, accessed 13 December 2013).

[43] National AIDS Authority. Costs and cost-effectiveness of HIV prevention and impact mitigation interventions in Cambodia. Phnom Penh: UNAIDS; May 2012 (http://www.aidsdatahub.org/sites/default/files/documents/Cost_effective_HIV_prevention_interventions_2012.pdf, accessed 13 December 2013).

[44] National Center for HIV/AIDS, Dermatology and STDs. Cambodia 2007 Behavioral surveillance survey. Phnom Penh: NCHADS; 2007 (http://www.nchads.org/Publication/BSS/Behavioral%20Surveillance%20Survey%20Cambodia-2007.pdf, accessed 13 December 2013).

[45] Cambodia country progress report. Monitoring the progress toward the implementation of the Declaration of Commitment on HIV and AIDS (January 2010–December 2011). Phnom Penh: National AIDS Authority; 2012 (http://www.unaids.org/en/dataanalysis/knowyourresponse/countryprogressreports/2012countries/ce_KH_Narrative_Report%5b1%5d.pdf, accessed 13 December 2013).

[46] National Center for HIV/AIDS, Dermatology and STDs. Standard operating procedures for HIV, STI and TB-HIV prevention, care, treatment and support in prisons (and correctional centres) in Cambodia. Phnom Penh: Ministry of Interior and Ministry of Health; January 2012 (http://www.nchads.org/SOPs/SOP%20for%20Prison%20Setting%20Eng.pdf, accessed 12 November 2013).

[47] Gardner EM, McLees MP, Steiner JF, del Rio C, Burman WJ. The spectrum of engagement in HIV care and its relevance to test-and-treat strategies for prevention of HIV infection. Clin Infect Dis. 2011;52:793–800. doi: 10.1093/cid/ciq243.

[48] Standard operating procedure for implementation of the boosted linked response between HIV and SRH for elimination of new paediatric HIV infections and congenital syphilis in Cambodia. Phnom Penh: National Center for HIV/AIDS, Dermatology and STDs; April 2013 (http://www.nchads.org/index.php?id=21, accessed 12 November 2013).

[49] Standard operating procedure for the boosted continuum of prevention, care and treatment for most-at-risk populations in Cambodia. Phnom Penh: National Center for HIV/AIDS, Dermatology and STDs; 2013 (http://www.nchads.org/index.php?lang=en, accessed 12 November 2013).

[50] Concept note on treatment as prevention (TasP) as a strategy for elimination of new HIV infections in Cambodia. Phnom Penh: National Center for HIV/AIDS, Dermatology and STDs; 2012.

[51] Framework for metrics to support effective treatment as prevention. Meeting report. Geneva: World Health Organization; 2012. (http://www.who.int/hiv/pub/meetingreports/framework_metrics/en/index.html, accessed 12 November 2013).

[52] National Center for HIV/AIDS, Dermatology and STDs. HIV/AIDS and STI prevention and care programme. Comprehensive report, third quarter 2012 (http://www.nchads.org/Report/q3_Comp_Report_2012%20eng.pdf, accessed 12 November 2013).

[53] National Center for HIV/AIDS, Dermatology and STDs. Annual report 2011. Phnom Penh: Ministry of Health; 2012 (http://www.nchads.org/Report/Annual%20Report%202011%20Eng.pdf, accessed 12 November 2013).

[54] National Center for HIV/AIDS, Dermatology and STDs. Standard operating procedures for HIV testing and counselling "HTC". 2012. (http://www.nchads.org/index.php?lang=en, accessed 12 November 2013).

[55] Standard operating procedures (SOP) to initiate a linked response for prevention, care, and treatment of HIV/AIDS and sexual and reproductive health issues. Phnom Penh: Ministry of Health; 2007 (http://www.nchads.org/SOPs/SOP%20to%20Initiate%20a%20link%20respose%20en.pdf, accessed 12 November 2013).

[56] Delvaux T, Samreth S, Barr-DiChiara M, Seguy N, Guerra K, Ngauv B et al. Linked response for prevention, care, and treatment of HIV/AIDS, STIs, and reproductive health issues: results after 18 months of implementation in five operational districts in Cambodia. J Acquir Immune Defic Syndr. 2011;57:e47–e55.

[57] Medley A et al. Maximizing the impact of HIV prevention efforts: interventions for couples. AIDS Care. 2013;25:1569–80.

References

[58] National Center for HIV/AIDS, Dermatology and STDs. Fourth quarterly comprehensive report, 2012. Phnom Penh: Ministry of Health; 2012 (https://www.nchads.org/Report/q4_2012_compr_report%20en.pdf, accessed 12 November 2013).

[59] National Center for HIV/AIDS, Dermatology and STDs. Continuum of care for people living with HIV/AIDS in Cambodia: operational framework. Phnom Penh: Ministry of Health; 2003 (http://www.nchads.org/AIDS%20Care/CoC%20framework%20English.pdf, accessed12 November 2013).

[60] National Center for HIV/AIDS, Dermatology and STDs. Standard operating procedure for implementing MMM activities in Cambodia. Phnom Penh: Ministry of Health; 2006. (http://www.nchads.org/SOPs/\\SOP%20for%20MMM%20(ENG).pdf, accessed 13 December 2013).

[61] Thai S, Koole O, Un P, Ros S, De MP, Van Damme W et al. Five-year experience with scaling-up access to antiretroviral treatment in an HIV care programme in Cambodia. Trop Med Int Health. 2009;14:1048–58.

[62] National Institute of Statistics, Directorate General for Health, and ICF Macro. Cambodia Demographic and Health Survey 2010. Phnom Penh, Cambodia and Calverton, Maryland, USA: National Institute of Statistics, Directorate General for Health, and ICF Macro; 2011 (http://www.measuredhs.com/pubs/pdf/FR249/FR249.pdf, accessed 12 November 2013).

[63] National Institutes of Statistics, Ministry of Planning Cambodia and Directorate General for Health, Ministry of Health. Demographic and health survey 2010. Calverton, Maryland: Measure DHS; September 2011 (http://www.unicef.org/cambodia/Cambodia_DHS_2010_Complete_Report_Part1.pdf, accessed 13 December 2013).

[64] Isaakidis P, Raguenaud ME, Te V, Tray CS, Akao K, Kumar V et al. High survival and treatment success sustained after two and three years of first-line ART for children in Cambodia. J Int AIDS Soc. 2010;13:11. doi: 10.1186/1758-2652-13-11.

[65] Janssens B, Raleigh B, Soeung S, Akao K, Te V, Gupta J et al. Effectiveness of highly active antiretroviral therapy in HIV-positive children: evaluation at 12 months in a routine program in Cambodia. Pediatrics. 2007;120(5):e1134–40.

[66] National Center for HIV/AIDS, Dermatology and STDs. National guidelines for the use of antiretroviral therapy in adults and adolescents. Second revision. Phnom Penh: Ministry of Health; 2012 (http://www.nchads.org/Guideline/National%20Guidelines%20%20for%20the%20use%20ART%20for%20adults%20and%20adolescents%202012%20Eng.pdf, accessed13 November 2013).

[67] Antiretroviral therapy for HIV infection in adults and adolescents: recommendations for a public health approach: 2010 revision. Geneva: World Health Organization; 2010 (http://www.who.int/hiv/pub/arv/adult2010/en/, accessed13 November 2013).

[68] National Center for HIV/AIDS, Dermatology and STDs. Annual report 2010. Phnom Penh: Ministry of Health; 2011 (http://www.nchads.org/Report/annual%20report%202010%20eng.pdf, accessed 20 December 2013).

[69] Ferradini L, Ouk V, Segeral O, Nouhin J, Dulioust A, Hak C et al. High efficacy of lopinavir/r-based second-line antiretroviral treatment after 24 months of follow up at ESTHER/Calmette Hospital in Phnom Penh, Cambodia. J Int AIDS Soc. 2011;14:14.

[70] Nerrienet E, Nouhin J, Ngin S, Segeral O, Ken S et al. (2012) HIV-1 protease inhibitors resistance profiles in patients with virological failure on LPV/r-based 2nd line regimen in Cambodia. J AIDS Clinic Res. 2012;S5:003. doi: 10.4172/2155-6113.S5-003

[71] Ministry of Health, Royal Government of Cambodia. National strategy for reproductive and sexual health in Cambodia: 2006–2010. Phnom Penh: Ministry of Health; 2008 (http://www.moh.gov.kh/files/mch/NSRSH%202006-2010.pdf, accessed 13 December 2013).

[72] Global tuberculosis report 2012. Geneva: World Health Organization; 2012 (http://apps.who.int/iris/bitstream/10665/75938/1/9789241564502_eng.pdf , accessed 13 December 2013).

[73] Guidelines for intensified tuberculosis case-finding and isoniazid preventive therapy for people living with HIV in resource-constrained settings. Geneva: World Health Organization; 2011 (http://www.who.int/tb/challenges/hiv/ICF_IPTguidelines/en/index.html, accessed 13 December 2013).

[74] World Health Organization. External quality control system (EQAS). (http://www.who.int/gfn/activities/eqas/en/, accessed13 November 2013).

[75] National Strategic Plan for Blood Transfusion Services, 2013–17, Phnom Penh: Ministry of Health; 2013.

[76] International Monetary Fund.. World Economic Outlook Database. 2013. (http://www.imf.org/external/pubs/ft/weo/2013/02/weodata/index.aspx, accessed 13 December 2013).

[77] International Labour Office. Cambodia Social Protection and Public Expenditure Review. EU/ILO Project on "Improving Social Protection and Promoting Employment" In cooperation with the GIZ Social Health Protection Programme, Cambodia, in the context of the P4H initiative. Geneva: International Labour Office; 2012 (http://www.ilo.org/wcmsp5/groups/public/---ed_protect/---secsoc/documents publication/wcms_secsoc_34870.pdf, accessed 15 December 2013).

[78] National Centre for HIV/AIDS, Dermatology, and STDs, National AIDS Authority, and Joint United Nations Programme on HIV/AIDS. National AIDS Spending Assessment IV. Prepared by Anastasiya Nitsoy. Phnom Penh: 2013.

[79] Costing HIV/AIDS in Cambodia: improving unit cost data. Draft prepared by Lawrence Seale and Anastasiya Nitsoy. Phnom Penh: US Centers for Disease Control and Prevention and Joint United Nations Programme on HIV/AIDS; 2013.

[80] National AIDS Authority. Costs and cost-effectiveness of HIV prevention and impact mitigation interventions in Cambodia. Phnom Penh: 2012 (http://www.aidsdatahub.org/costs-and-cost-effectiveness-of-hiv-prevention-and-impact-mitigation-interventions-in-cambodia-national-aids-authority-cambodia-2012, accessed 15 December 2013).

Annex I: Review team members

External review team
- **Daniel Tarantola**, MD, Ferney-Voltaire, France, Review team leader
- **Richard Steen**, BS in Health Sciences, MPH, Middlesex, Vermont, United States
- **Polin Chan**, MD, Master of Epidemiology, Vaux-Chavanne, Belgium
- **Nick Walsh**, MD, Phnom Penh, Cambodia
- **Ron Wherens**, MSc in Pharmacy, MBA, PK Ankeven, Netherlands
- **Jerry Owen Jacobson**, BS, MPhil. Policy Analysis, PhD., Bogata, Columbia

External secretariat team
- **Ying-Ru Lo,** MD, Team Leader HIV & STI, WHO Regional Office for the Western Pacific, Manila, the Philippines
- **Annie Chu**, ScD, Health Economist, WHO Regional Office for the Western Pacific, Manila, the Philippines
- **Nathan Shaffer**, MD, PMTCT Lead, WHO Headquaters, Department of HIV/AIDS, Geneva, Switzerland
- **Suman Jain**, MBBS, MPH, Monitoring and Evaluation, The Global Fund to Fight AIDS, Tuberculosis and Malaria, Geneva, Switzerland
- **Ryuichi Komatsu**, MD, Monitoring and Evaluation, The Global Fund to Fight AIDS, Tuberculosis and Malaria, Geneva, Switzerland

Local review team, Phnom Penh, Cambodia
- **Seng Sopheap**, MD, National Center for HIV/AIDS, Dermatology and STDs (NCHADS) (Policy, Strategies, STI control)
- **Mok Sokuntheary**, MD, NCHADS (Monitoring and Evaluation)
- **Sau Sokunmealiny**, MD, NCHADS (Strategic Information)
- **Seng Vuthy**, MD, NCHADS (HIV Care and Treatment)
- **Tuon Sovanna**, MD, National Maternal and Child Health Center (NMCHC) (PMTCT, Linkages)
- **Khun Kim Eam**, MD, National Center for Tuberculosis and Leprosy Control (CENAT), (TB/HIV, Linkages)
- **Prom Chanrith**, Team Leader for Planning, Monitoring and Reporting at KHANA
- **Ly Vanthy**, MD, US CDC expert (Community and Health System Strengthening)
- **Lam Phirun**, MD, Reproductive Health Programme, NMCHC (Sexual and Reproductive Health)

Local secretariat team
- **Seng Sopheap**, MD, NCHADS
- **Mok Sokuntheary**, MD, NCHADS
- **Masami Fujita**, MD, WHO Cambodia
- **Marie-Odile Emond**, UNAIDS Cambodia
- **Dora Warren**, MD, Centers for Disease Control and Prevention, Global AIDS Programme (CDC GAP), Cambodia

Local steering committee

Mean Chhi Vun, MD, Director, NCHADS	Chair
Ly Penh Sun, MD, Deputy Director, NCHADS	Alternate Chair
Daniel Tarantola, MD, HIV Review Team Leader	Co-Chair
Khun Kim Eam, MD, CENAT	Member
Tuon Sovanna , MD, NMCHC	Member
Ngin Lina, MD, Director, Department of Planning, Monitoring and Evaluation, National AIDS Authority	Member
Ly Vichea Ravuth, MD, Depart of Planning and Health Information	Member
Masami Fujita, MD, Local Secretariat Team	Member
Sedtha Chin, UNICEF	Member
Marie-Odile Emond, Local Secretariat Team	Member
Oum Sopheap, MD, KHANA	Member
Emily Welle, Clinton Health Access Initiative (CHAI)	Member
Laurent Ferradini, MD, FHI 360	Member
Sorn Sotheariddh, Cambodian People living with HIV/AIDS Network (CPN+)	Member
Chan Dyna, entertainment worker network c/o Cambodian Women for Peace and Development (CWPD)	Member
Lor Seyha, men who have sex with men/ transgender networks	Member
Taing Phoeuk, people who use drugs/ people who inject drugs (PWUD/PWID)	Network
Dora Warren, MD, US CDC, Local Secretariat Team,	Member
Saba Moussavi, The Global Fund HIV SSF Project	Member
Robin Martz, USAID	Member
Suos Premprey, MD, AusAID	Member
Seng Sopheap, MD, NCHADS, Local Secretariat Team	Secretary
Mok Sokuntheary, MD, NCHADS, Local Secretariat Team	Secretary

Annex II: Overall schedule, scope and process of national health sector review

This paper highlights key features of the health sector review of the national programme against HIV/sexually transmitted infections (STIs). It incorporates information drawn from various documents that have set out the purpose and objectives of the review (which are not repeated here). The present paper extends this information by adding details on the scope of the review.

This document assumes that the national health sector review of the response to HIV/STIs in Cambodia will take place from 29 April to 10 May 2013.

A. Scope of the review

The topics listed below may be considered for inclusion in the agenda of the national health sector HIV/STI review. However, this list should be significantly reduced so as to make the review more focused and manageable, and less of a burden on the national staff. Within each of the topics retained eventually for the programme review, one or more specific issues of importance should be chosen and a specific question asked. The review method and instruments will then be designed to best respond to the question raised.

> Applicable to all items listed below is seeking and documenting the evidence of strengths, weaknesses, successes, shortcomings, gaps and opportunities for strategic improvements through better use of available data, resources and research.

(1) **Status and trends of HIV/AIDS and STIs, and their impact on individuals, communities and society:**
- Validity and robustness of epidemiological data (biological and behavioural HIV and STI surveillance and periodic surveys, HIV case reports, STI case reports), subpopulation size estimates and data reflecting the cascade of access to and provision of health services
- Trends in stigma and discrimination related to HIV and/or key-affected populations such as sex workers, men who have sex with men, transgender people and people who inject drugs
- Strengthening production and analysis of outcome and impact data
- Use of data for programme and service improvement

(2) **Policy, strategy, management and coordination arrangements, including community engagement:**
- Level of political commitment and whether the health sector response is embedded in an overall multisectoral response to HIV/STIs
- Level and quality of community engagement in prevention and care of HIV and other STIs
- Patterns of education, training and employment of human resources for health engaged in HIV/STI work; advisability and feasibility of a performance-based incentive scheme; prevention and mitigation of high staff turnover, workload and burn-out
- Awareness of HIV-related policies, laws and strategies among health personnel at different levels of the health system
- Awareness of relevant policies, laws and strategies among civil authorities
- Assessment of relevance, adequacy, coherence and adherence of governmental and nongovernmental organizations (NGOs) to national HIV-related policies, laws and strategies
- Collaboration with NGOs/civil society organizations (CSOs): extent, quality, efficiency, sustainability and mutual accountability
- Action at the community level: special attention to key affected populations and ensuring sustained HIV awareness and engagement of rural, urban and mobile communities
- Gender- and age-specific needs and gaps

(3) **Prevention, HIV testing and counselling, care and treatment:**
- Performance of current interventions/services
- HIV treatment as a prevention strategy
- Management of dual HIV/TB infection
- Quest for a synergy between prevention, care and treatment
- Diagnostic HIV testing: partner and couples testing
- Boosted Continuum of Prevention to Care and Treatment (CoPCT) among key-affected populations
- Follow up after HIV testing, linkages to care and treatment (treatment metrics)
- Community outreach services
- Demand for, access to, and use of condoms
- Demand for, access to, and use of clean injecting equipment
- Social networks relevant to HIV/STIs (e.g. key-affected populations, young people, migrants)
- Institutionalized populations (e.g. prisons and other closed settings)
- Provider-initiated HIV and syphilis testing in antenatal care and in the community, uptake of antiretrovirals (ARVs) for prevention of mother-to-child transmission (PMTCT) and how to transition to Option B+
- Post-exposure prophylaxis after accidental occupational exposure for health-care workers and accidental sexual exposure and rape; HIV and reproductive choices

(4) Procurement and laboratory issues of HIV and STI testing, and treatment and care monitoring
- Procurement and supply management systems for laboratory supplies and equipment, pharmaceuticals, logistics and communication as part of broader health systems capacity enhancement
- Access to, coverage and quality assurance of HIV testing (voluntary counselling and testing, and provider-initiated testing and counselling), and STI and tuberculosis (TB) diagnoses
- Access to and quality of biological monitoring of antiretroviral therapy (ART)
- Early detection of treatment failure, ARV resistance and indications for ART regimen changes

(5) Strategic and management information systems
- Performance of the strategic and management information system
- Recording, reporting and data analysis at national, institutional, regional, district and local levels
- Strengthening data production and management to inform and support strategic investments for impact
- Mapping populations at higher HIV risk and vulnerability (entertainment workers and male and female sex workers, people who use drugs, men who have sex with men, transgender people, mobile populations)
- Advisability and feasibility of introducing a unique identifier in the data management system, completeness, timeliness, robustness and use of HIV, STI, TB/HIV and behavioural surveillance data
- Drug resistance surveillance
- Information sharing (e.g. TB) and dissemination

(6) Linkages: both with and within the public and private health sector
- National Health Strategic Plan, 2008–2014
- Maternal and child health
- Primary health care
- Malaria
- Reproductive and sexual health
- TB
- Noncommunicable diseases
- Health information system
- Occupational health
- Law enforcement agencies and other uniformed personnel
- Links to other sectors of development

(7) National AIDS Spending Assessment (NASA) and attribution of outcome and impact
- Analysis of the cost of the programme and services, and national AIDS expenditures
- Attribution of HIV/STI programme outcomes and impacts to investments

(8) Health systems and sustainable financing
- Current patterns and predictable trends, supply and gaps in national and international financing of the health sector response to HIV/STI
- Internal and external accountability on resource use
- Identification of sustainable financing mechanisms

Specific questions for the programme review arising from the January 2013 impact review:
(1) How to operationalize the cascade of services from prevention to treatment?
(2) What should be the performance measure of outreach activities – from information, testing to case detection, linkage to care and treatment?
(3) What are and should be the supporting environment measures for activities among key-affected populations?
(4) What empirical evidence can/should inform prioritization of services, including costing, mapping, population size?
(5) How to improve linkages with the health system, including decentralization, maternal and child health, TB, health worker incentives?

The national health sector HIV/STI review report should clearly identify the achievements and strengths, weaknesses, gaps and challenges, and make recommendations for consolidating and improving programme effectiveness.

B. Review process

PREPARATORY PHASE I (March 2013)
- Establish a Steering Committee
  - The Steering Committee would be established specifically for the health sector review of the national response to HIV/STIs and related infections.
  - It could consist of about 12 members, including representatives of NCHADS and of other suitable departments of the Ministry of Health (MOH); representatives of international partners (WHO, Global Fund, UNAIDS); delegate(s) from NGOs dedicated to HIV; representative(s) of people living with HIV and other members of civil society; and the external chair of the review team.
- Designate a programme review Secretariat.
- Hold an initial meeting of the Secretariat to agree on procedures for the preparation of the first Steering Committee meeting and documents to be tabled at that meeting.
- Hold an initial preparatory meeting of the Steering Committee to:
  - define and agree to the purpose of and set objectives for the review, and determine the optimal process for the review and finalization of the report;
  - stimulate general support for the review and access to stakeholders' information; and
  - prepare desk reviews on different topics (epidemiological data, monitoring data, other documents and reports).

- Hold a second Secretariat meeting to agree on a consolidated set of review objectives, dates, schedule and review team members, and begin the process of selecting geographical areas and institutions to be visited by the review team.
- Consolidate the list of sites/institutions to be visited by the review team. These could include, for example:
  - At the national level:
    - an initial presentation by the leadership of NCHADS to the review team (also to be invited to be present should be the executive heads of national health services and of the TB programme;
    - one or two hospitals with the heaviest HIV case load (adults and children);
    - one or two obstetric departments with the heaviest case load in PMTCT;
    - the executive heads of the departments responsible for maternal and child health, sexual/reproductive health; planning; pharmaceutical and non-pharmaceutical procurement;
    - the national HIV reference laboratory;
    - a prison and a closed setting, e.g. rehabilitation centre where key populations, people living with HIV may be detained;
    - key unilateral and multilateral organizations engaged in HIV work;
    - key NGOs engaged in HIV work with a focus on key populations;
    - project sites serving entertainment workers with a large number of clients, injecting drug users, men who have sex with men and transgender people; and
    - transgender people.
  - At the peripheral level:
    - three provincial headquarters and provincial hospitals outside Phnom Penh with prime responsibility for HIV/STI. Judging by existing reports and observations by central staff, one of these could be a province considered as performing well, another as performing poorly and yet another as performing at an average level. Apart from meeting with health staff and visiting health-care facilities, the review team should also call on local administrative authorities for reasons of courtesy and to seek their views on HIV in their area of responsibility. Selected NGOs engaged in HIV work should also be forewarned of the visit and invited to present their projects to the review team.
    - in each of these provinces, three districts could be chosen for visits by the review team: one judged to have a high performance, another with average performance and a third with low performance relative to the overall performance of the province.
    - within each of these districts, two communities served by subdistrict health facilities could be selected for site visits: one with good access to and use of HIV services, the other with poor or no access to or use of services.
- Altogether, the review team would visit three provinces (in addition to Phnom Penh), nine districts and 18 communities. In order to avoid excessive preparation in the selected provincial, district and local sites, it would be preferable to inform the authorities at these sites only three to four weeks ahead of the visits.

PREPARATORY PHASE II (April 2013)

- Subsequent meetings of the review Secretariat should be concerned with administrative and logistic arrangements, including the following:
  - finalization of a day-by-day schedule for the review team (to be consolidated in consultation with the co-leaders of the review);
  - logistic arrangements for site visits (a transportation coordinator; transportation could be by government vehicles, hired taxis or local car-rental private companies);
  - administrative arrangements (preparation and dispatch of introductory materials to be provided to team members; reservation of a meeting room and equipment; access to internet and photocopying services; reservation of accommodation; designation of one or two English-speaking secretarial staff; and
  - financial matters (budget preparation, purchase of fuel, collection of receipts for local expenditures to cover per diem and petty cash for some local expenses by national staff).
- The co-leaders of the review team and Secretariat will develop instruments for data collection, consolidation and analysis by review team members. These will draw from instruments used in other countries in the Region and adapted to best suit the Cambodian reality. Review methods and instruments will also draw on materials produced by WHO, UNAIDS and the Global Fund, as well as other trusted sources as the need arises.
- The preliminary schedule, review method and instruments will be sent by the Secretariat to members of the review ream.
- The data collection instruments designed for the provincial and district levels should be tested in one province and one district. This province and district should not have been selected for the actual review.

CONDUCTING THE REVIEW (29 April–10 May 2013)

- All review team members should be present in Phnom Penh on the eve of the starting date of the review. The review will formally begin in the morning of Monday 29 April (Day 1) but documents and last minute instructions may be made available to review team members the night before.
- Day 1 (Monday 29 April): review team meeting, clarification of review objectives and individual schedules. Presentations by central team, preparation for stakeholder meeting
- Day 2 (Tuesday 30 April): stakeholder meeting, open to all registered institutions and persons engaged in HIV/STI work. This may be a 90-minute meeting at which the objectives, schedule and methods of the review will be presented. Comments and suggestions to make provincial-, district- and subdistrict-level visits more effective will be invited. The rest of the day will be used to familiarize review team members with the review methods and instruments. The review team will be divided in four sub-teams (three for provincial and district visits, one to remain in Phnom Penh).
- Day 3 (Wednesday 1 May): national holiday. Compilation of documents, finalization of review methods and instruments, travel to sites for field teams
- Days 4–5 (Thursday 2 May–Friday 3 May): the review team is divided in four sub-teams (three for provincial and district visits, one to remain in Phnom Penh) for further visits to official development agencies, international NGOs, NGOs and central institutions and departments of the MOH. Each sub-team is composed of a national and an external review team member accompanied by a staff of NCHADS fluent in English, who can work as a translator and a contact person with the NCHADS Central Office.

- Days 6–7 (Saturday 4 May–Sunday 5 May): all sub-teams travel back to Phnom Penh on Saturday: team meeting on Sunday to take stock of work done and check if any information gap needs to be filled. Compilation of data, reading, drafting contributions to the report
- Days 8–10 (Monday 6 May–Wednesday 8 May): Consolidation of inputs by review team members to a preliminary executive summary accompanied by a set of recommendations to be submitted to national and international authorities invested in the review for a first reading. Follow-up visits to institutions and programme or project sites can be arranged during these two days but these should be scheduled outside slots of time that will be set aside for meetings of sub-teams or the whole team.
- Day 11 (Thursday 9 May): presentation of preliminary review findings to stakeholders, inviting comments
- Day 12 (Friday 10 May): presentation of preliminary report to the MOH authorities and feedback session/workshop to discuss the review findings with people engaged in HIV work.

FOLLOW UP (11 May–10 June)
- Consolidation of a full draft report and review by team members
- Submission of a revised full report to organizations invested in the review
- Final editing and dissemination of the full report.

C. Review team

Review team members are acting in their personal capacity and do not represent formally the institution to which they may be affiliated. They should have no conflict of interest with the review role they are invited to perform. They will be made aware that no reprimand or sanction will be addressed to individuals or groups as a result of the findings arising from the review. Part-time participation in the review or observer status will be strongly discouraged as this has proved to be extremely disruptive in other settings.

All review team members (national and external) should be able to communicate efficiently in English and be available for the whole duration of the review, including for travel within the country. **National review team members** can be drawn from within the MOH or from other sectors as long as they are sufficiently familiar with the national response to HIV/STIs. They can be chosen from the private health sector or from the local NGO community or other members of civil society. **External review team members** will be nominated and recruited by WHO in consultation with other entities invested in the review.

The review team will have two co-leaders (one national, the other external), plus nine national and nine external members (to be nominated). One or more team members should have expertise in each of the following fields:
- HIV surveillance
- HIV and TB with a focus on TB and HIV/TB surveillance
- Logistics and procurement supply management
- Strategic and management information
- STI and key populations
- PMTCT/maternal and child health/sexual and reproductive health
- PMTCT and paediatrics
- HIV and hepatitis coinfections, harm reduction
- Care and ART
- Asia Pacific Network of Positive People (APN plus)
- Blood safety, safe injections and clinical technology
- Health financing.

D. Background documents to be made available to the review team

All documents made available to members of the January 2013 outcome and impact review should be made available to the programme review team through a freshly created Dropbox. In addition, the following documents should be dropped in that box:
- the summary and performance framework of ongoing agreements with the Global Fund
- the WHO/Global Fund draft guide for conducting national programme reviews of the health sector response to HIV
- global Fund evaluation approach and definitions
- global Fund monitoring and evaluation assessment checklist
- a link to the UNAIDS website where various guidelines for monitoring and evaluation can be accessed, in particular, concerning prevention among key populations. (http://www.unaids.org/en/data analysis/datacollectionandanalysisguidance/monitoringandevaluationguidelines/).
- the list of documents will be adjusted as the review agenda becomes more focused.

Annex

Annex III: Programme of work and assignments

1. Programme areas and methods

Five programme areas identified by the Steering Committee
(1) Policy, strategy and service delivery
(2) Strategic information
(3) Health financing, including national AIDS spending assessment (will be conducted before the mission, no expert identified)
(4) Linkages, health systems strengthening, and community systems strengthening
(5) Procurement and supply management and laboratory

Methods
- Semi-structured questionnaires during interviews and focused group discussions with stakeholders, including civil society representatives, clients and patients
- All teams will cover the overall review questions plus specific additional thematic areas according to the team members' expertise.

Writing assignments
The team was assigned writing tasks. Daniel Tarantola, Jerry Jacobson, Richard Steen, Ying-Ru Lo were members of the core writing team. All review team members wrote sections pertaining to their specific areas of expertise.

2. Mission Programme

Programme

Time	Topic	Venue/Institution /Address	Team
Friday, 26 April–Saturday, 27 April: Final preparations			
12:00 onwards	Final preparations for review	WHO	Daniel Tarantola, Ying-Ru Lo Core group of Steering Committee
Sunday, 28 April 2013			
16:00–18:00	Introductions and briefing by team leader	Hotel The Plantation, Phnom Penh	External team
18:00	Review of documents		External team
Monday, 29 April 2013			
	Introductions, purpose, objectives of review	Hotel The Plantation, Phnom Penh	Steering Committee Local and external team External Secretariat
	Review methodology		
	Review draft tools and questionnaires		
	Review documents		
Tuesday, 30 April 2013			
09:00–17:00	Stakeholder meetings and site visits in Phnom Penh	Hotel Himawari, Phnom Penh	All teams (See programme in Annex IV)
Wednesday, 1 May 2013			
	Travel to the field and site visits in Phnom Penh	Battambang Province Svay Rieng Province Banteay Meanchey Province Phnom Penh	All teams (See programme in Annex IV)

Programme

Time	Topic	Venue/Institution/Address	Team
Thursday, 2 May 2013			
	Field visits	Continued	See schedule for field visits
Friday, 3 May 2013			
	Field visits	Continued	See schedule for field visits
Saturday, 4 May 2013			
	Return from field visits		
Sunday, 5 May 2013			
	Writing individual assignments	Hotel The Plantation, Phnom Penh	
Monday, 6 May 2013			
	Site visits in Phnom Penh for last-minute visits and collection of information needed	Phnom Penh	Selected external team members
	Review team meeting: consolidation of findings	Hotel The Plantation, Phnom Penh	
Tuesday, 7 May 2013			
	Team reports by field visit	Hotel The Plantation, Phnom Penh	Last-minute visits and collection of additional information needed
	Review team meeting: consolidation of findings		
	Writing provisional report		
Wednesday, 8 May 2013			
	Review team meeting: consolidation of findings	Hotel The Plantation, Phnom Penh	
	Writing provisional report		
Thursday, 9 May 2013			
	Team reports by thematic area and writing	Hotel The Plantation, Phnom Penh	
Friday, 10 May 2013			
	Meeting with H.E. The Minister of Health	Chamber of the Minister	
	Stakeholder meeting and validation workshop	Phnom Penh hotel	
Saturday, 11 May 2013			
	Finalization of draft executive summary	Hotel The Plantation, Phnom Penh	Writing team

Annex

Annex IV: Meetings and visits to institutions in Phnom Penh
26 & 30 April and 6-7 May 2013

The below schedules do not include all ad hoc and site visits to local partners and institutions.

Group assignment			
Group I	**Group II**	**Group III**	**Group IV**
Programme area: Policy, strategies, systems, financing, linkages, blood safety, TB/HIV, MCH	Programme area: Strategic information	Programme area: Maternal Child Health (MCH), PMTCT, HIV testing and counseling Team	Programme area: HIV prevention, closed settings
Seng Sopheap	Mok Sokuntheary	Lam Phirun	Seng Vuthy
Ly Vanthy	Prom Chanrith	Tuon Sovanna	Khun Kim Eam
Polin Chan	Sau Sokun Mealiny	Ayesha de Lorenzo	Richard Steen
Ron Wherens	Jerry Owen Jacobson	Ying-Ru Lo	Nick Walsh
Annie Chu	Suman Jain	Nathan Shaffer	Daniel Tarantola
	Dora Warren	Masami Fujita	Marie-Odile Emond

30 April 2013

Group 1

Time	Key informants	Venue	Team involved
14:00–15:00	United States Government Agencies	United States Agency for International Development (USAID), Centers for Disease Control and Prevention (CDC) Global AIDS Program, President's Emergency Plan for AIDS Relief	III
15:30–17:00	Australian Agency for International Development (AusAID)	AusAID	III

Group 2

Time	Key informants	Venue	Team involved
14:00–15:00	National AIDS Authority (NAA)	NAA	II
15:30–17:00	National Authority for Combating Drugs (NACD)	NACD	II

Group 3

Time	Key informants	Venue	Team involved
14:00–15:00	Global Fund Principal Recipient, Ministry of Health (MOH)	MOH	I
15:30–17:00	Department of Planning and Health Information	MOH	I

Group 4

Time	Key informants	Venue	Team involved
14:00–15:00	General Department of Prison (GDP), Ministry of Interior	GDP	IV
15:30–17:00	One prison in Phnom Penh	Site visit	IV

6 May 2013

Group 1

Time	Key informants	Venue	Team involved
08:00–09:00	Global Fund Prinicipal Recipient, National Center for HIV/AIDS, Dermatology and STDs (NCHADS): Data Management Unit (DMU)	NCHADS	I
10:30–12:00	PR-NCHADS: Logistics Management Unit (LMU), Procurement	NCHADS	I
14:00–15:00	Local Fund Agent (LFA)	LFA	I
15:30–17:00	Populations Services International (PSI)	PSI	I

Group 2

Time	Key informants	Venue	Team involved
08:00–09:00	National Programme of Mental Health, MMT Clinic	Mental Health Programme	IV
10:30–12:00	Department of Health, Ministry of Interior	Department of Health, MOH	IV
14:00–15:00	Men's Health Cambodia (MHC)	MHC	IV
15:30–17:00	Needle and syringe programme (NSP) site Outreach visit	Field visit	IV

Group 3

Time	Key informants	Venue	Team involved
08:00–09:00	National Centre for Tuberculosis and Leprosy Control (CENAT)	CENAT	II
10:30–12:00	National Maternal and Child Health Centre (NMCHC)	NMCHC	II
14:00–15:00	National Blood Transfusion Center (NBTC)	NBTC	II
15:30–17:00	NCHADS laboratory	NCHADS	II

Group 4

Time	Key informants	Venue	Team involved
08:00–09:00	University of Health Sciences (UHS)	UHS	III
10:30–12:00	School of Nursing	School of Nursing	III
14:00–15:00	School of Public Health	NIPH	III
15:30–17:00	National Institute of Public Health (NIPH) laboratory	NIPH	III

Annex

7 May 2013

Group 1

Time	Key informants	Venue	Team involved
08:00–09:00	FHI 360	FHI 360	II
10:30–12:00	Chouk Sar 1&2 Clinics	Site visit	II
14:00–15:00	Smart-Girl network Outreach visit	Site visit	II
15:30–17:00	M-Style network Outreach visit	Site visit	II

Group 2

Time	Key informants	Venue	Team involved
08:00–09:00	KHANA	KHANA	IV
10:30–12:00	Cambodian People Living with HIV/AIDS Network (CPN+)	CPN+	IV
14:00–15:00	ARV Users Association (AUA)	AUA	IV
15:30–17:00	Reproductive Health Association of Cambodia (RHAC)	RHAC	IV

Group 3

Time	Key informants	Venue	Team involved
08:00–09:00	Department of Drug and Food (DDF), Ministry of Health	MOH	I
10:30–12:00	Central Medical Store (CMS)	CMS	I
14:00–15:00	Reproductive and Child Health Alliance (RACHA)	RACHA	I
15:30–17:00	UNICEF Chief of Supply section	UNICEF	I

Group 4

Time	Key informants	Venue	Team involved
08:00–09:00	Cambodian Women for Peace and Development (CWPD)	CWPD	III
10:30–12:00	National Paediatric Hospital (NPH)	NPH	III
14:00–15:00	Kossamak Hospital	Kossamak Hospital	III
15:30–17:00	Chamkardong pre-ART/ART site	Chamkardong Hospital	III

Annex V: Summary of recommendations

The review team concluded that the Cambodian response to HIV was progressing well towards its 2011–2015 strategic objectives, and that it was on track for eliminating the transmission of HIV by 2020 if the following conditions are met:

- Structures, capacities and services dedicated to HIV and STI prevention, care and treatment, and the early diagnosis and treatment of HIV/TB coinfection are further strengthened and sustained

- Access to services by the most vulnerable and key-affected populations (including entertainment workers, female and male sex workers, men who have sex with men, transsexual and transgender persons and drug users) is expanded and, in some cases, revitalized in a supportive legal and policy environment.

- Stronger follow up is conducted along the cascade of services, from creation of and demand for voluntary HIV testing and counselling to sustained and efficiently monitored use of care and treatment, devoting particular attention to gender issues, age and key-affected populations. These efforts could be considerably strengthened through effective and better strategic information management, linkage of databases, and tighter communication and collaboration among service providers.

- Sharper epidemiological targeting and more effective interventions are introduced at sufficient intensity and scale to identify new HIV infections and treatment introduced earlier to harness the dual benefit of mortality reduction and prevention of further spread of HIV among those at highest risk.

- Access to, and voluntary use of, HIV counselling and testing by pregnant women attending antenatal clinics is expanded, with full and timely provision of antiretroviral therapy for life during pregnancy and/or shortly before delivery to protect offspring from HIV infection.

- Stronger synergy is fostered within the health sector and across other sectors of development.

- Greater support is provided to health personnel through improved salary, skills upgradation and incentives to ensure staff retention. The health of the Cambodian population is ensured and protected against brain drain and the loss of those who care for them.

- Sustained external financing is assured and a growing financial share secured from national sources.

The review team formulated a series of specific recommendations which, if implemented with a sustained sense of urgency and bolstered by the needed human and financial resources, should enable Cambodia to achieve elimination of new HIV infections by 2020.

1. Policy, strategy and structures

1.1 The alignment about to begin within the MOH departments and initiatives may be arranged in a way that it generates synergies, with expanded benefits accruing to all concerned programmes, while protecting and nurturing their respective gains.

1.2 During 2013–2014, it is suggested that a feasibility assessment be carried out and a roadmap drawn to further adapt the role and functions of NCHADS to (i) the evolving HIV/STI situation, (ii) the strategic changes reflected in the new conceptual framework, and (iii) the health sector capacity in the country. Till the assessment is done, it would be best to preserve the structure, management and staff of NCHADS at the present level.

1.3 By actively pursuing the development of operational plans of the Cambodia 3.0 framework, NCHADS would be taking advantage of the opportunity to remedy the fragmentation of programme strategies resulting from an ever-expanding series of interventions. Interventions, related standard operating procedures and performance monitoring could be consolidated in the form of a compact, outcome-driven programme informed by evidence.

1.4 By the end of 2014, the MOH would have developed its change strategy in consultation with other partners within the health sector and funding agencies. The MOH could then engage with determination in a transition towards more effective linkages on HIV across concerned departments and initiatives within the health sector and with external partners. While NCHADS would remain the backbone of the national response to HIV and STIs in the near future, it is important that it play a central role in the elaboration and unfolding of the change strategy in its domain of activity.

1.5 Given the alarming trends in staff shortages and turnover, there is an urgent need to reinforce the human resources capacity in the formal health sector. The recently produced definition of roles and tasks of NCHADS is an important step in this direction. The review team recommends that, within the MOH, the Department of Human Resources under the Directorate General for Health and the Department of Personnel under the Directorate of Administration and Finance jointly formulate a plan to respond to this pressing issue.

1.6 The salary scale and associated incentives offered to the health workforce should match the current economic reality in Cambodia, and ensure that the retention and good performance of the human resources engaged in combating HIV STI are valued and protected. The review team urges the Minister of Health, the Council of Administrative Reform and higher authorities to deal with this matter urgently. Failing to do so may lead to further degradation of the livelihood and morale of health staff, and impede the performance of the system.

1.7 Strengthening the interaction between the NAA and NCHADS would be beneficial. The review team took note of the upcoming mid-term review of the multisectoral strategic plan on HIV undertaken by the NAA. In order to avoid duplication of efforts, this review agreed not to cover the health sector. The review team recommends that the outcome of the present health sector's response to HIV be considered in the broader multisectoral review, and that, in return, the findings of the review of the multisectoral response to HIV inform the health sector's response to HIV so as to create mutually beneficial synergies.

1.8 It is suggested that the MOH, through NCHADS, ensure that the recommendations contained in this report are translated into an operational plan, implemented with the needed support and followed up.

2. Creating an enabling environment

Assessing and adjusting harmful policies and laws

2.1 The creation of an enabling environment for the response to HIV requires that the benefits and risks associated with every policy enacted by any branch of the government be assessed from a dual HIV and public security perspective before being promulgated. The method of health impact assessment could be used to project the possible impact of proposed new policies and laws on HIV. This method is increasingly being applied in the South-East Asia and Western Pacific regions.

2.2 Implementation of existing and planned initiatives such as the Police–Community Partnership Initiative designed to strengthen enabling environments should receive high priority under the Boosted Continuum of Prevention to Care and Treatment, and be adequately monitored and periodically assessed against their intended outcomes.

2.3 The MOH should make the health workforce more familiar with the 2002 HIV law. It is important to retrain health staff in providing services and being responsive to thespecial needs of men, women and children living with HIV. It would also be helpful to provide opportunities for health workers to express their fears rationally and fulfil their obligations professionally through group discussions in which peers and people living with HIV should participate.

3. Strategic information

Surveillance: keeping pace with an evolving epidemic

3.1 It is recommended that strategies by which surveillance studies in risk groups could be strengthened to improve upon city-/provincial-level estimates, especially for larger cities and those areas with the greatest epidemic burden, be assessed by a national working group on HIV strategic information. Evaluating different options would help to ensure that the most critical information is collected at minimal cost.

3.2 It is recommended that trend analysis of the sociodemographic and behavioural characteristics of individuals who test positive for HIV at voluntary counselling and testing sites be included in their programme reports. It needs to be explored whether such trends can best be ascertained by analysis of individual-level databases or by introducing HIV case reporting (i.e. individual-level instead of aggregate-level reporting) with confidentiality protections. Given the likelihood of underreporting of stigmatized risk behaviours, data from voluntary counselling and testing sites should be triangulated with other data sources, such as data from outreach programmes and surveillance studies.

3.3 Current efforts are warranted by NCHADS and partners to assess the feasibility of using routine data from PMTCT programmes instead of unlinked, anonymous HIV testing for surveillance purposes. Issues to be explored include the level of agreement of prevalence estimates between data from routine PMTCT services and unlinked, anonymous HIV testing at antenatal clinic facilities; the impact of selection bias on prevalence estimates using PMTCT programme data; and the potential impact of using service-based data for surveillance purposes on attendance at antenatal clinic services.

3.4 It is recommended that analyses be developed to assess trends in HIV incidence based on trends in prevalence among young antenatal attendees <24 years (or <20 years if the data allow) and incidence trends determined in integrated biological and behavioural surveillance studies by newly developed assays.

Mapping and estimating the size of key-affected populations

3.5 It is suggested that current efforts continue by NCHADS and partners to standardize methods for mapping and size estimation of key-affected populations. A national plan is recommended to ensure that estimates are reliable and updated regularly (every two years). The plan would need to define methods for both mapping (as a part of routine programme management) and population size estimation (derived from mapping and surveillance surveys) for the population in each city/province, with standard definitions and timelines. It is recommended that efforts to strengthen programmatic data quality and use these in conjunction with surveys to develop the size estimates be included in the plan. As improved methods become available (every three to four years), it is suggested that the existing methods be reviewed and revised.

3.6 NCHADS can play an important role by providing technical guidance, in coordination with nongovernmental organizations and community members, and by ensuring that a mechanism is in place to provide regular training and technical supervision during data collection. Allowing for technical input from local academic institutions may prove useful.

3.7 In order to improve the set of size estimates available for all risk groups, it is recommended that additional methods such as the "unique object" and "unique event" methods in conjunction with surveys be explored.

Monitoring the quality of HIV programmes

3.8 Potential gains in efficiency could be explored by consolidating the CQI and EWI indicators in a single set of quality-monitoring indicators and by unifying analysis, training and follow-up functions under one NCHADS unit to avoid duplication. It is suggested that CQI's unique emphasis on CoC team meetings and follow up be retained under the new, consolidated system. While technically distinct, if the findings from cohort analysis are made available more regularly to CoC teams, they can be reviewed together with the quality indicators, thus providing a more complete picture of trends in patient outcomes.

3.9 It is suggested that a plan with concrete steps to decentralize analysis to the provincial health department and operational district be developed, with increased training and coordination by NCHADS and phased roll-out, beginning with high-burden areas.

3.10 A mechanism to regularly review existing evidence of loss to follow up along the services cascade is recommended in order to develop targeted qualitative assessments to identify reasons for loss to follow up. Assessments may focus on links in the cascade where existing evidence indicates potential problems.

Monitoring linkages along the services cascade: the need for a unique identifier

3.11 NCHADS' efforts to develop a combination of unique identifier systems across the continuum of prevention, care and treatment services are well founded. Establishing well-defined criteria to guide discussion among stakeholders and the eventual selection of a method for introducing a combination of unique identifier systems is recommended.

3.12 The review team wishes to draw the attention of the MOH, NCHADS, service providers and civil society to the need for ensuring the protection of privacy and confidentiality, along with the creation of complaint and redressal mechanisms. These mechanisms should be prepared to respond to possible breaches of confidentiality of personal data, as new data management systems are being designed for the purpose of tracking people living with HIV throughout the continuum of prevention, care and treatment.

3.13 It is recommended that profiles of the epidemic and response be developed and regularly updated (annually) through greater and integrated analysis of data from surveillance studies, routine surveillance, community outreach and health services. Characterizing recent changes in the epidemic situation, particularly with respect to new HIV and STI infections, and effectiveness of the response will provide stakeholders with the information they need to improve the targeting of interventions. Both national- and local-level profiles need to be considered. A phased roll-out, beginning with profiles for the highest-burden regions or cities/provinces, is recommended.

4. Maintaining control of the epidemic

Sharper epidemiological targeting

4.1 Outreach and services to drug-injecting women and drug-injecting men who have sex with men and transgender persons in Phnom Penh and other identified urban areas should be prioritized within the Boosted Continuum of Prevention to Care and Treatment strategy as a first step to ensuring high coverage of these key populations. Ensuring a more enabling environment and peer/community engagement is critical to the success of these efforts.

4.2 NCHADS should consider establishing an

Annex

epidemiological rapid response mechanism following the principles of standard communicable disease outbreak investigation and control, with resources to investigate pockets of potential high incidence (HIV, STI and related infections), and to quickly strengthen the response in such areas.

Entertainment workers

4.3 The Boosted Continuum of Prevention to Care and Treatment strategy should strengthen outreach activities that intensify interventions for subpopulations of entertainment workers at greatest vulnerability and risk. These population include (i) entertainment workers with a large number of sexual partners (more than seven partners a week), (ii) entertainment workers at venues where sex takes place on site (quasi-brothels, guesthouses, massage parlours, etc.), (iii) drug-using entertainment workers and (iv) non-establishment-based entertainment workers in settings of potential high vulnerability (streets, truck stops, etc.).

4.4 In addition to the above, it is recom-mendended that hidden high-transmission sex work networks be investigated through formative and intervention-linked research, utilizing peer networks and proven epidemiological methods (snowball sampling, rapid response methods, etc.).

Men who have sex with men and transgender persons

4.5 Existing interventions with men who have sex with men should be strengthened under the Boosted Continuum of Prevention to Care and Treatment strategy. Focusing on men who sell sex and men in non-paying "pleasure circuits" (frequenting saunas, for example) with large numbers of partners, as well as drug-using men who have sex with men is suggested. Strengthening the link to STI services (for routine check ups and syphilis screening) would help to control the rising incidence of ulcerative STIs in this population. (Monitoring the rising incidence of STIs acts as an indicator of the effectiveness of prevention efforts.)

4.6 Outreach and peer interventions to trans-gender persons, especially those who use drugs, along with appropriate services and follow up, are an immediate priority, while more complete mapping, size estimates and biobehavioural data on higher-risk subpopulations are carried out to guide the response.

People who use drugs

4.7 It is recommended that the MOH, through the National Program of Mental Health, NCHADs and other relevant partners scale up the coverage of needle–syringe programmes and related services to people who inject drugs across Phnom Penh, utilizing secondary needle–syringe programme distribution (through networks of people who inject drugs) and working with local authorities to improve access and reach hidden populations.

4.8 Scale up methadone maintenance treatment programmes within Phnom Penh to ensure wider coverage. It would be advisable to focus initially on rapidly expanding the existing service service while maximizing retention in treatment provision of take-home dosing, and lowering the threshold for drop-outs who restart treatment.

Closed settings

4.9 The Ministry of Interior, through the General Department of Prisons, should introduce HIV prevention interventions, including the provision of condoms, as a priority in closed settings. For prison inmates who inject drugs, it is suggested that harm reduction including opioid substitution therapy be made available, with referral to services in the community on release from prison, ensuring continuity of care for those on opioid substitution treatment.

4.10 Considering the commendable introduction of active TB case-finding in closed settings, the review team recommends the offer of provider-initiated voluntary HIV testing and counselling by all prison health posts to prison inmates, as described in the 2012 Standard operating procedures for HIV, STI and TB/HIV prevention, care, treatment and support in prisons (and correctional centres) in Cambodia. It is advised that ART, isoniazid preventive therapy, TB and STI treatment (in accordance with national standard operating procedures) be provided to all coinfected patients. Infection control measures would also need to be introduced and prison personnel trained accordingly.

STI services

4.11 The national network of STI clinics, which performs a critical prevention function for key-affected populations, should be reinforced. In order to ensure user-friendliness and unimpeded access to services, upgradation of services would be needed. NCHADS could upgrade and consider expanding the STI services (Family Health Clinics), strengthening capacity and increasing user-friendliness and access for key-affected populations. Building the capacity of Family Health Clinics would help them to function as the local "eyes" of the "rapid response mechanism" (*see* recommendation 4.2), and take an active role in monitoring "hotspots" and community-based interventions, investigating outbreaks and strengthening the response.

4.12 Strengthening the analysis and use of routine STI

data is needed to pinpoint areas where increasing STI rates indicate that the prevention response may be weak, and this information could be used to inform the work of the rapid response mechanism described above. Information obtained from new male STI patients about venues of recent sexual exposure could be used to strengthen prevention work in those areas.

4.13 It is recommended that the role and performance of STI control in the overall response to HIV be reviewed. Strengthening the capacity for STI control is advised in targeted prevention efforts (through routine check-ups of entertainment workers, men who have sex with men and transgender persons), routine monitoring and surveillance of sexual transmission trends. Priority indicators for prevention of sexual transmission would need to include trend analysis of male STI case reports (genital ulcers and urethral discharge), as well as monitoring of syphilis prevalence and incidence among entertainment workers, men who have sex with men and transgender persons.

5. **Optimizing the cascade of interventions: HIV testing, linkages to prevention, care and treatment**

Earlier diagnosis of HIV status and enrolment to care

5.1 Ongoing efforts to decentralize HIV testing (first screening test) and train peer outreach workers, health centre and maternal and child health staff including midwives in conducting voluntary counselling and HIV testing should continue in order to make available same-day test results, link individuals into care and follow them through treatment. Quality management systems will have to be expanded to include community-based testing.

5.2 It is advised that maternal and child health services and NCHADS continue to offer HIV testing to male partners and family members, including children of HIV-positive pregnant women in antenatal settings, and consider expansion of this offer to HIV-positive index persons receiving voluntary counselling and testing and OI/ART care. Putting in place systems to monitor uptake of such testing and linking test results, for example, of partners of HIV-positive index persons, would facilitate intensified HIV prevention for serodiscordant couples.

5.3 The concept of "shared confidentiality" could be considered for application by NCHADS in health-care settings. This would need to be tested and implemented with utmost caution, and monitored and protected. It is advisable for trained health-care workers within and across health facilities from health centre to referral hospital to be aware of the HIV status, co-morbidities and clinical treatment of their patients. This information could be made available to trained treatment supporters with the consent of the client. Likewise, information on follow up of people living with HIV by the MMM and other self-help groups could be made available to health staff in the same facility to ensure the continuum of care.

5.4 For consenting clients, the role of treatment supporters could be expanded to involve selected trained prevention outreach workers who work with specific key populations (for example, HIV-positive men who have sex with men) to ensure retention in care. As in health-care facilities, this would need to be tested and implemented with utmost caution, and monitored and protected.

5.5 As recommended by WHO, a focused strategy should be developed of re-testing those with indeterminate results (a positive screening test but not confirmed) or those with higher risk rather than re-testing every individual with a negative test result.

Care and treatment for adults, adolescents and children

5.6 Ongoing efforts to update the 2012 national ART guidelines and the 2012 concept note on "treatment as prevention" in line with the new 2013 WHO guidelines should continue. An evaluation after one year of the change in threshold for starting ART and ability to implement that change, as well as the effect on median CD4 count at start of ART would help inform Cambodia 3.0. Increasing access to ART for key-affected populations is an immediate priority.

5.7 Ongoing effort to phase out d4T and introduce TDF for adults, adolescents and children should continue. Ensuring appropriate and adequate procurement and supply of TDF and paediatric formulations to treat the range of age- and weight-band groups according to guidelines is an important improvement in HIV care for adults and children.

5.8 NCHADS may consider improving the existing mechanisms to support and promote adherence and retention, and minimize loss to follow up through task-sharing as a part of decentralization of treatment. This could include a review of the current scheme with MMM and enhancing coordination at all levels to fit into the current needs of the national programme and the 3.0 strategy. For example, active case management could be done by trained people living with HIV, drawn from health centres, MMM groups of people living with HIV or peer outreach workers, and the role of ART counsellors expanded to serve as case managers to help staff at the ART clinics. This would strengthen the interface between facility, community and home-based care.

5.9 Strengthening institutional capacity would be important for providing paediatric and adolescent HIV care, including age-appropriate disclosure of HIV status to the child and adolescent, addressing emerging sexuality needs during adolescence and young adulthood, as well as transitioning to adult services. Renewed focus on the "family continuum of care" would support the 3.0 strategy.

5.10 It is suggested that further assessment of paediatric and adolescent HIV care and treatment, including for HIV-exposed infants, incorporate an analysis of the data from various cohorts to understand the quality of paediatric and adolescent care services, and whether current recording and reporting systems are equipped to provide data useful for the programme.

5.11 Linking NCHADS with maternal and child health services is advised for offering other care services, including sexual and reproductive health, family planning and cervical cancer screening for women living with HIV and female entertainment workers. Emerging co-morbidities from noncommunicable diseases due to the prolonged provision of ART may also be considered.

Prevention of mother-to-child transmission (PMTCT) of HIV

5.12 The standard operating procedures for the Boosted Linked Response by both NMCHC and NCHADS support PMTCT Option B+. It is recommended that implementation of these standard operating procedures be actively pursued, and the relevant documents disseminated to district and health centre levels (not just at the provincial level).

5.13 NCHADS and NMCHC should develop clear targets for both coverage and final outcome measures for 2015. It would also be necessary to calculate annual mother-to-child transmission rates based on the cohort data from PMTCT programmes and infant outcomes through 2020, for both ART and maternal and child health.

5.14 The PMTCT programme may consider a routine offer of combined screening for haemoglobin, HIV, syphilis and hepatitis testing to pregnant women attending antenatal care, as part of basic antenatal screening, and monitor its uptake.

5.15 It is suggested that enhanced linkages among the current data systems of the maternal and child health programme and NCHADS be established so that subset analysis could be performed for the needs of each programme, e.g. ART in pregnant women and infants/children/adolescents.

5.16 A situation analysis may be considered to review private sector involvement in HIV services.

Monitoring the cascade

5.17 Regular use of different types of data including routine programme data to understand the patient cohort and provide data for decision-making, assess programme performance and address bottlenecks along the cascades at national and subnational levels is recommended.

5.18 Impact analysis and evaluation of outcomes could be strengthened, as they are critical to inform whether algorithms and interventions are working.

6. Tuberculosis and HIV

6.1 The HIV review team endorses the recommendations on TB/HIV made by the joint TB programme review in 2012 and their implementation.

6.2 Efforts to reduce TB deaths among people living with HIV will require enhanced efforts, not only for HIV case detection and provision of co-trimoxazole prophylaxis and ART, but also for active case detection of TB, and provision of isoniazid preventive therapy and TB treatment among people living with HIV.

6.3 Current efforts at active TB case-finding in closed settings should be complemented by the systematic offer of HIV testing and further expansion of TB infection control measures.

6.4 Establishing a corresponding computerized electronic TB programme database could help harmonization of data collection, validation and analysis at all levels of services across the two programmes.

6.5 It is advised that TB diagnosis among people living with HIV using Xpert MTB/RIF be expanded nationwide as soon as possible.

7. HIV/STI laboratory services

7.1 In order to oversee, supervise, build capacity and monitor overall HIV/STI laboratory capacities, it is recommended that national reference laboratories be strengthened. Enhancing the laboratories would entail the strengthening of human resources, technology and coordination between apex services. It is suggested that the patient information systems on early infant diagnosis be strengthened so that the records of mother and infant pairs are linked. Ideally, the early infant diagnosis database would be linked to the patient monitoring database of NCHADS and PMTCT.

7.2 As recommended in the 2013 WHO treatment guidelines, NCHADS should consider investing more in viral load monitoring, and set reasonable goals for 2015 and 2020 to allow appropriate planning for resource needs. Engaging with partners would help NCHADS to think about how best to utilize CD4 counts in a changing environment.

7.3 It is recommended that coverage of the EQAS programmes for HIV and STI antibody testing be sustained and cover the full array of tests in all facilities providing HIV testing. These would include HIV and syphilis rapid tests, validation of HIV testing algorithms using rapid tests, CD4 count and viral load, as well as early infant diagnosis.

7.4 Innovative diagnostic approaches, including point-of-care CD4 counts, and point-of-care molecular diagnostic platforms such as GeneXpert® for HIV viral load, chlamydia and gonorrhoea may be considered.

7.5 It is advised that existing STI surveillance be strengthened with periodic etiological studies and gonococcal antimicrobial resistance monitoring (GASP) to support STI case management.

8. Pharmaceutical supply management

8.1 NCHADS' approach to national fore-casting for ARVs is sound, but the methodology used, including responsibilities, data flow, assumptions and timings, needs to be better documented and informed by evidence and experience. Doing so would help reduce the Global Fund's anxiety over possible misquantification and, therefore, speed up order approvals. The method would need to take into account the longer lead times of the voluntary pooled procurement mechanism and set appropriate safety stock levels.

8.2 NCHADS may consider engaging a laboratory specialist to develop a documented method for, and lead the forecasting and monitoring of, HIV diagnostics/laboratory supplies.

8.3 NCHADS may continue using voluntary pooled procurement to procure pre-qualified ARVs and other large-value items at competitive prices in compliance with the Global Fund procurement rules. However, alternative mechanisms acceptable to the Global Fund need to be identified to procure the wide range of OI/STI medicines, HIV diagnostics and laboratory consumables required by the programme in smaller quantities. Options could be an agreement with an international wholesaler or with UNICEF.

8.4 It is suggested that NCHADS and USAID-funded RACHA collaborate towards integrating NCHADS Excel-based ordering system into the HOSDID system used for essential drugs. This may require a switch from the current patient-based order system to an average consumption approach. While the RACHA system may require some site-specific adjustments, especially for less commonly used products such as second-line ARVs, the system is robust enough to handle the majority of needed supplies. Doing so would reduce the workload at the NCHADS Local Management Unit, which can then focus on more strategic national forecasting challenges.

9. Blood safety

9.1 The review team endorses the recommendations made by the 2012 comprehensive assessment of blood transfusion services, and supports their early implementation.

9.2 The National Blood Transfusion Center may consider strengthening procurement and supply management of test kits for TTIs (HIV, hepatitis B virus, hepatitis C virus, syphilis), in line with recommendation 8.2.

9.3 The National Blood Transfusion Center, NCHADS and the National Reference Laboratory are advised to strengthen coordination to ensure EQAS for test kits in the programme, in line with recommendation 7.3.

10. Sustainable financing for the HIV/AIDS response

10.1 For informing priority-setting and maximizing value for money to serve as key inputs to the multi-year strategic plan, it would be necessary to generate and use evidence. The strategic plan would have to include a resource needs and mobilization plan. The programme could increase value for money by allocating resources to the most effective programmes and improving service delivery and management efficiencies in informing the prioritization of essential HIV/AIDS services for its resource needs and mobilization plan, given its absorptive capacity.

10.2 It is important to routinely monitor and evaluate the funding and expenditure levels, resource allocations and efficiency of the programme, including how to gradually increase linkages with other entities in the health system.

10.3 Domestic funding can be increased through supply- (e.g. ARVs, condoms, HIV testing) and demand-side financing (e.g. inclusion of ART, STI services in social health protection schemes). It is important to assess mechanisms to achieve this as part of emerging developments in Cambodia's health financing policy to move towards universal health coverage.

10.4 NCHADS should be actively involved and engaged in the development of the Cambodia health strategic plan and health financing policy, which are in the early stages of development. These measures will constitute a major step towards long-term sustainability and expanded linkages of the HIV programme to the health system.